Basic Laparoscopy
&
Instrumentation

Video Contents

1. Diagnostic Laparoscopy with Adhesiolysis

2. Laparoscopy Appendicectomy

3. Laparoscopic Cholecystectomy

Basic Laparoscopy & Instrumentation

Second Edition

Sadashiv Patil
MS FMAS FIAGES FACRSI
Professor
Department of General Surgery
Sapthagiri Institute of Medical Sciences
Bengaluru, Karnataka, India

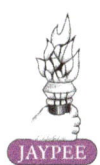

JAYPEE BROTHERS MEDICAL PUBLISHERS
The Health Sciences Publisher
New Delhi | London

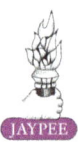

Jaypee Brothers Medical Publishers (P) Ltd

Headquarters
Jaypee Brothers Medical Publishers (P) Ltd
EMCA House, 23/23-B
Ansari Road, Daryaganj
New Delhi 110 002, India
Landline: +91-11-23272143, +91-11-23272703
+91-11-23282021, +91-11-23245672
Email: jaypee@jaypeebrothers.com

Corporate Office
Jaypee Brothers Medical Publishers (P) Ltd
4838/24, Ansari Road, Daryaganj
New Delhi 110 002, India
Phone: +91-11-43574357
Fax: +91-11-43574314
Email: jaypee@jaypeebrothers.com

Overseas Office
JP Medical Ltd.
83, Victoria Street, London
SW1H 0HW (UK)
Phone: +44 20 3170 8910
Email: info@jpmedpub.com

EU GPSR Authorised Representative
Logos Europe, 9 rue Nicolas Poussin
17000, La Rochelle, France
Phone: +33 (0) 6 67 93 73 78
E-mail: Contact@logoseurope.eu

Website: www.jaypeebrothers.com
Website: www.jaypeedigital.com

© 2025, Jaypee Brothers Medical Publishers

The views and opinions expressed in this book are solely those of the original contributor(s)/author(s) and do not necessarily represent those of editor(s) or publisher of the book.

All rights reserved. No part of this publication may be reproduced, stored or transmitted in any form or by any means, electronic, mechanical, photocopying, recording or otherwise, without the prior permission in writing of the publishers.

All brand names and product names used in this book are trade names, service marks, trademarks or registered trademarks of their respective owners. The publisher is not associated with any product or vendor mentioned in this book.

Medical knowledge and practice change constantly. This book is designed to provide accurate, authoritative information about the subject matter in question. However, readers are advised to check the most current information available on procedures included and check information from the manufacturer of each product to be administered, to verify the recommended dose, formula, method and duration of administration, adverse effects and contraindications. It is the responsibility of the practitioner to take all appropriate safety precautions. Neither the publisher nor the author(s)/editor(s) assume any liability for any injury and/or damage to persons or property arising from or related to use of material in this book.

This book is sold on the understanding that the publisher is not engaged in providing professional medical services. If such advice or services are required, the services of a competent medical professional should be sought.

Every effort has been made where necessary to contact holders of copyright to obtain permission to reproduce copyright material. If any have been inadvertently overlooked, the publisher will be pleased to make the necessary arrangements at the first opportunity.

Inquiries for bulk sales may be solicited at: jaypee@jaypeebrothers.com

Basic Laparoscopy & Instrumentation

First Edition: 2016

Second Edition: **2025**

ISBN: 978-93-5696-747-2

Dedicated to

Parents, Wife and Son

Preface to the Second Edition

Laparoscopy and endoscopy are established in urban areas to a large extent. Still, they have to penetrate the rural areas.

We already know the advantages of laparoscopy such as small scar, reduced surgical site infection, less pain, early recovery, early return to work, minimal loss of blood and cosmetics. The disadvantages are steep learning curve for the Doctor, loss of hand-eye coordination, 2D image, change in ergonomics.

Focus needs to be changed to learn laparoscopic skills, taking this into consideration I have added one new chapter, i.e., Endotrainer and made changes to chapter of Ergonomics.

This book is handy, simple language and affordable. After reading the book, young upcoming surgeons can upgrade their knowledge.

Sadashiv Patil

Preface to the First Edition

We have seen that there was exponential growth of endoscopy and laparoscopy, in particular, in the last two to three decades. In recent times, no other field of medicine has grown as fast as this. There are some great advantages of laparoscopy such as minimal pain, minimal blood loss, faster recovery, minimal loss of working days and cosmesis. The disadvantages are loss of hand-eye coordination and technically demanding.

Though it has grown exponentially, there is a need for it to penetrate the rural areas. This book is written particularly keeping in mind the young upcoming surgeons and postgraduates. After reading this book, the rural surgeons can practice basic laparoscopy in rural areas.

I have been practicing laparoscopy since 15 years and have also read some books in laparoscopy written by international and Indian national. These books provide insights in the field of laparoscopy, but affordability is difficult due to high price. That is why I felt the need to write this book, *Basic Laparoscopy & Instrumentation*, which should be at affordable price.

I hope that this book will generate some interest in the field and will be of some benefit to the upcoming surgeons.

Sadashiv Patil

Acknowledgments

Many thanks to my parents, wife and son, and other members of my family on this occasion for bringing out this book, *Basic Laparoscopy & Instrumentation*, for their patience, love and affection.

I would also like to thank St John's Medical College, Bengaluru, Karnataka, India, where I am working as Associate Professor. My special thanks to the Dean and the management for helping me to publish this book. I would take this opportunity to thank my seniors in the department along with the juniors, friends and the librarian.

I take this opportunity to thank Shri Jitendar P Vij (Group Chairman), Mr Ankit Vij (Managing Director), Priyansh Saxena (Development Editor), and all the staff of Bengaluru Production Unit of M/s Jaypee Brothers Medical Publishers (P) Ltd, New Delhi, India.

Contents

1. **Beginning of Laparoscopy** 1
   - History *1*

2. **Imaging System in Laparoscopy** 7
   - Camera *7*
   - Laparoscope *8*

3. **Instruments** 13
   - Laparoscopic Hand Instruments *13*

4. **Pneumoperitoneum** 24
   - Insufflators *24*
   - Terminologies *25*
   - Pneumoperitoneum Insufflation *26*

5. **Peritoneal Access** 30
   - Anatomy of Anterior Abdominal Wall *30*
   - Methods of Peritoneal Access *30*

6. **Electrocautery** 36
   - Newer Energy Sources *36*

7. **Harmonic and Vessel Sealing Device** 43
   - Ultrasonic Shears (Harmonic) *44*
   - Bipolar Vessel Sealing Device *45*

8. **Homeostasis and Suturing** 47
   - Homeostasis and Suturing Technique *47*

9. **Troubleshooting and Complications** 56
   - Troubleshooting in Laparoscopy and Remedies *56*
   - Complications of Laparoscopy *57*

10. **Laparoscopic Appendectomy** 60
    - Appendicitis *60*
    - Laparoscopic Appendectomy *63*

11. Anatomy and Physiology of Gallbladder ... 67
- Surgical Anatomy of Gallbladder 67
- Surgical Physiology of Gallbladder 69

12. Chronic Cholecystitis ... 71
- Natural History 71

13. Acute Cholecystitis ... 73
- Clinical Features 73
- Treatment 74
- Acalculous Cholecystitis 74

14. Laparoscopic Cholecystectomy ... 76
- History of Cholecystectomy 76
- Operative Setup 77
- Port Positions 77
- Procedure 79

15. Diagnostic Laparoscopy ... 87
- Procedure 87
- Indications 87

16. Ergonomics in Laparoscopic Surgery ... 94
- Mechanics and Principal Angles 94
- Instruments 95
- Principles of Port Placement 96
- Operating Room Environments 97

17. Endotrainer ... 100
- Components 100
- Suturing Exercises 101
- Endotrainer Exercises 101

Index ... 105

CHAPTER 1

Beginning of Laparoscopy

■ HISTORY

The beginning of the modern endoscopic/laparoscopic era is the early 19th century when Phillip Bozzini[1] described a cystoscope (1805).

The changes in surgical endoscopy leading up to 1988 were, in fact, gradual and evolutionary. For any major change or progress to take place, many factors must fall into place. In the case of laparoscopy, dramatic technical innovations were required. Momentum always favors inertia. Fears must be overcome, i.e. fear of making mistakes; fear of failure; fear of established procedures becoming obsolete and fear of established authorities losing control. Successful change requires timing and a force more powerful than the status quo.

Georg Kelling

On September 23, 1901, Georg Kelling, a surgeon and gastroenterologist, performed a laparoscopy on a live dog in front of an audience at the 73rd Congress of the Naturalist Scientist's Medical Conference, in Hamburg, Germany (Fig. 1.1). He named the procedure 'coelioscopy' (also spelled coelioskopie or koelioskopie). During Kelling's demonstration of a laparoscopy using a live dog as a subject, he made an incision through which he inserted a Nitze-Leiter cystoscope to magnify and view inside the abdomen.

The Nitze-Leiter cystoscope, first used in 1872, created illumination through an electrically heated platinum wire that allowed Kelling to see the interior of the abdomen through telescopic lenses. He then created a second incision, placing a trocar in the abdomen to insufflate the cavity with air, which allowed a better visual. This event marked the first laparoscopic endeavor. The dog survived the procedure. After performing coelioscopy on 20 dogs, Kelling deemed the procedure safe, noting that after an examination, a dog is as cheerful as it was before (the procedure).

Hans Christian Jacobaeus

Hans Christian Jacobaeus (Fig. 1.2), a Swedish internist, performed clinical laparoscopic surgery on a human—an electrical worker who had been diagnosed with hepatic cirrhosis.[2] Unlike Dr Kelling, Dr Jacobaeus did not use insufflations. Although not much is known about how Dr Jacobaeus

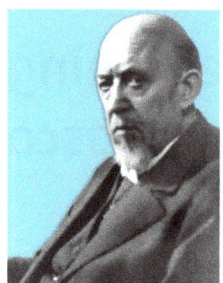

Fig. 1.1: Georg Kelling (1866–1945)

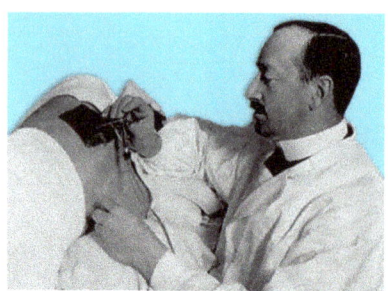

Fig. 1.2: Hans Christian Jacobaeus (1879–1937)

got involved in laparoscopic surgery, in 1912 he published a monograph describing the 97 laparoscopies he had performed between 1910 and 1912, in Stockholm's community hospital.[3] He observed that all of his patients, except one, improved after undergoing the procedure.

Bertram Bernheim

At almost the same time, Bertram Bernheim performed the first laparoscopic procedure in the United States at Johns Hopkins University Hospital, in 1911. He inserted a 12 mm proctoscope through an epigastric incision to inspect the peritoneal cavity in a jaundiced patient. In the following years, laparoscopy became an accepted diagnostic procedure. Because of its limited therapeutic applicability, the enthusiasm of general surgeons for the technique started to fade. Gynecologists became the users and advocates of this approach.

Zollikofer

Zollikofer, a Swiss gynecologist, introduced carbon dioxide to create pneumoperitoneum, in 1924 (instead of filtered air or oxygen, because of its fast absorption and to minimize the risk of explosion).

Heinz Kalk

In 1929, Heinz Kalk (Fig. 1.3), a German gastroenterologist developed a 135° lens system and used laparoscopy as a diagnostic method for liver and gallbladder diseases.

Kurt Semm

A German gynecologist, Kurt Semm (Fig. 1.4), then appeared on the scene. Born on March 23, 1927, in Munich, he attended Ludwig Maximilians University School of Medicine and received his degree in 1951, with a specialty in Obstetrics and Gynecology. He became fascinated with laparoscopy and explored the technique for almost 20 years before performing a laparoscopic appendectomy.

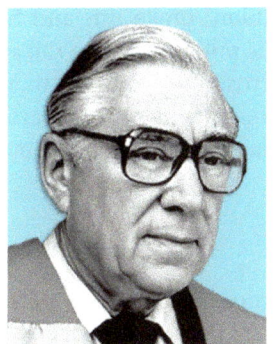

Fig. 1.3: Heinz Kalk

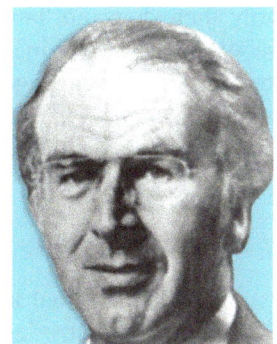

Fig. 1.4: Kurt Semm (1927–2003)

However, by the 1960s, laparoscopy had earned a bad reputation in Germany. It was associated with high complication rates, in part because surgeons were burning patients during laparoscopic procedures, so the technique was banned there temporarily. The ban was lifted in 1964.

By the late 1970s, doctors were performing a range of laparoscopic procedures, including myomectomy, ovariectomy, tubal ligation and ovarian cyst resection, and had helped to create new technologies such as the electronic insufflator (Figs 1.5 and 1.6).

In 1988, Semm traveled to Baltimore to present a video of his laparoscopic appendectomy. When Dr McKernan heard about this, he also traveled to Baltimore to view it. "Semm's procedure was on a horrible 8 mm film, but the second I watched it, I could see it involved basic surgical principles," he recalled. Intrigued, Dr McKernan returned home to Marietta, Georgia, to work on laparoscopy and shortly after he performed the first laparoscopic cholecystectomy in the United States. Dr McKernan said that "Semm is the Father of operative gynecology and he was so ahead of everyone else at that time".[4]

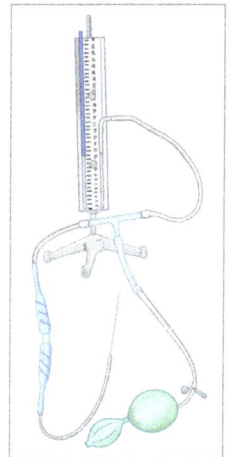

Fig. 1.5: Apparatus for creating Lufttamponade (Adapted from Schollmeyer, Mettler, Ruther, et al. Practical Manual for Laparoscopic and Hysteroscopic Gynecological Surgery, 2nd edition. 2013.)

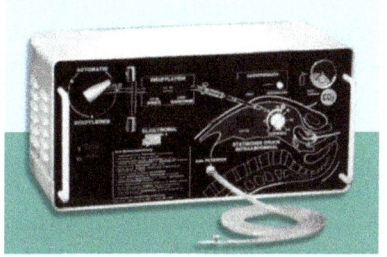

Fig. 1.6: Semm's electronic insufflator (Adapted from Semm K Endoscopy. 15(2);1983.)

Shortly thereafter, the 'laparoscopic revolution' broke out and Semm's laparoscopic expertise was in great demand. His publications on the subject, translated into many languages, were read across the world by thousands of surgeons. Without Semm's input, the development of a 'laparoscopic revolution', while perhaps inevitable, would have been postponed by many years.

Bosch/Power and Barnes

The first laparoscopic tubal ligation by electrocoagulation was performed in 1936 by Bosch in Switzerland, and in 1941 by Power and Barnes in Ann Arbor, Michigan. Scientific exchange during this time suffered because of the difficulties imposed by political agendas between World Wars.

Janos Veress

In 1938, the Hungarian physician, Janos Veress, developed a new needle for the creation of pneumothorax in patients with tuberculosis. Laparoscopists quickly realized the potential of using the needle in creating pneumoperitoneum with minimal risk of injuring intra-abdominal organs. The Veress needle has become the standard laparoscopic instrument ever since.[5] Zollikofer, a Swiss gynecologist, introduced carbon dioxide to create pneumoperitoneum in 1924 (instead of filtered air or oxygen because of its fast absorption and to minimize the risk of explosion).[6]

Harold Hopkins

After World War II, the discovery of the rod-lens system by Harold Hopkins and the cold light by Karl Stortz revolutionized laparoscopic imaging, and finally the laparoscopist could see clear and color-true images. More importantly, the risk of thermal injuries to the abdominal organs by incandescent light was eliminated.

Raoul Palmer

Raoul Palmer, the French gynecologist, changed the approach from the upper to the lower abdomen, placed his patient into the Trendelenburg position and stressed the importance of keeping the intra-abdominal pressure below 25 mm Hg.[6]

Philippe Mouret

In the late 1980s, laparoscopy was essentially a gynecologist's tool. One of the French private surgeon, Philippe Mouret of Lyon, shared his surgery practice with a gynecologist, and thus had access to both laparoscopic equipment and to patients requiring laparoscopy (Fig. 1.7). In March 1987, Mouret carried out his first cholecystectomy by means of electronic laparoscopy. Although he never published anything about this experience, the news on his technique reached Francois Dubois of Paris. The rapid acceptance of the technique of laparoscopic surgery by the general population is unparalleled in surgical history. It has changed the field of general surgery more drastically and more rapidly than any other surgical milestone. The technique of video laparoscopy popularized laparoscopic cholecystectomy around the world.

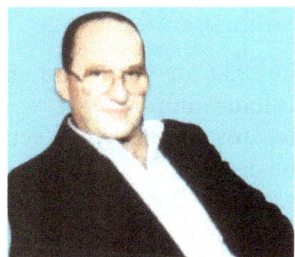

Fig. 1.7: Philippe Mouret

Francois Dubois

Although having no prior laparoscopic experience, Dubois acted immediately. He borrowed the instruments from gynecologists, performed his first animal experiments and, in April 1988, carried out the first laparoscopic cholecystectomy (LC) in Paris. Inspired by Dubois, Jacques Perissat of Bordeaux, introduced endoscopic cholecystectomy in his clinic and presented this technique at a Society of American Gastrointestinal Surgeons (SAGES) meeting in Louisville in April 1989. Very soon, news of the French work in LC soon swept beyond the country's borders. Dubois and Perissat spoke enthusiastically about their work at the meetings and were largely responsible for establishing what is today called the French technique.[7] It was not until after 1986, following the development of a video computer chip that allowed the magnification and projection of images onto television screens that the techniques of laparoscopic surgery truly became integrated into the discipline of general surgery.

National Institute of Health

The 1990s witnessed wide acceptance of laparoscopic surgery. In 1992, an National Institute of Health (NIH) conference declared that laparoscopic cholecystectomy should be the operation of choice for uncomplicated cholelithiasis.

Erich Mühe

In 1882, Carl Langebuch (1846-1901) of Germany performed the first cholecystectomy.[8] In 1985, Erich Mühe, a professor of surgery in Boblingen, Germany, used Semm's instruments and technique to remove the first gallbladder in the world, laparoscopically. Medicine made a tremendous leap forward in 1985 with the first laparoscopic cholecystectomy. The German Surgical Society rejected Mühe in 1986 after he reported that he had performed the first laparoscopic cholecystectomy, yet in 1992 he received their highest award, the German Surgical Society Anniversary Award.

Society of American Gastrointestinal Surgeons

In 1990, in Atlanta, at the SAGES convention, Perissat, Berci, Cuschieri, Dubois and Mouret were recognized by SAGES for performing early laparoscopic cholecystectomies, but Mühe was not. However, in 1999 he was recognized by SAGES for performing the first laparoscopic cholecystectomy and invited him to present the Storz lecture. In Mühe's presentation, titled 'The First Laparoscopic Cholecystectomy', which he gave in March 1999, in San Antonio, Texas, he described the first procedure. Finally, Mühe had received the worldwide acclaim that he deserved for his pioneering work.

REFERENCES

1. Kelley WE. The evolution of laparoscopy and the revolution in surgery in the decade of the 1990s. JSLS. 2008;12(4):351-7.
2. Jacobaeus HC, Ueber Die Moglichkeit, die Zystoskopic bei, Untersuching Seroser, Hohlungen anzuwenden, Vorlaufige Mitteilung. Germany: Münch Med Wochenschr; 1910. pp. 2090-2.
3. Jacobaeus HC. Über Laparo- und Thorakoskopie. Beitr Klin Tuberk. 1912;25: 185-354.
4. History of endoscopic and laparoscopic surgery. World J Surg. 1997;21(4):444-53.
5. Nezhat F. Triumphs and controversies in laparoscopy: the past, the present, and the future. JSLS. 2003;7(1):1-5.
6. Rosin D. History in minimal access medicine and surgery. Oxford, United kingdom: Radcliffe Medical Press; 1993. pp. 1-9.
7. Berci G. History of endoscopic surgery. In: FL Greene, JL Ponosky (Eds). Philadelphia: Saunders; 1994. pp. 1-5.
8. Victoria Stern. Laparoscopy: The Controversial Beginnings of a Surgical Revolution.

CHAPTER 2

Imaging System in Laparoscopy

CAMERA

Camera is an important component of imaging system. It is composed of charge-coupled device (CCD). CCD is an electronic device that is used to transfer electrical charge and it receives light as input. The CCD takes this optical input and converts it into an electronic signal—the output.

A CCD chip is a metal oxide semiconductor (MOS) device. Silicon is used as the base material and silicon dioxide is used as the coating material. The final, top layer is also made of silicon—polysilicon.

The word coupled is used in the CCD, because they are composed of array of imaging pixels and matching array of storage pixels that are coupled together. After an imaging array is exposed to light, its charges are quickly transferred to the storage array. While the imaging array is being exposed to the next picture, the storage array from the last picture are being converted to digital form by the analog to digital(A/D), converter a row at a time. The CCD converts the optical image into an electrical signal that is sent through the cable to the camera control unit (CCU).

Camera (Fig. 2.1) has two parts, head and the CCU (Fig. 2.2), which is located on the trolley. Single chip camera has one CCD for all colors whereas a three-chip camera has one CCD for each primary color red, green and blue.[1] Light is split into red blue and green by a prism present in the head of the camera.[2] The signals are picked by the sensors present on the CCD.[3]

White balancing has to be done in natural light, not under the over head lamp and white gauze is used for the same. Head is composed of a zoom lens that is used to focus the image. Focussing is done with suture material at a distance of 10 cm.

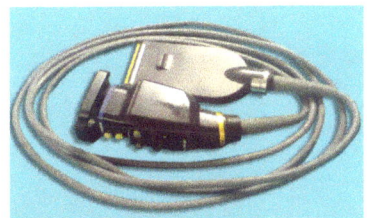

Fig. 2.1: Camera

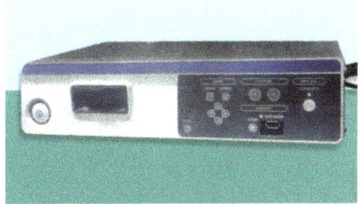

Fig. 2.2: Processor

LAPAROSCOPE

It was Jacobeans, who first referred to the word laparothorakoskopie when he published his work of inspection of the peritoneal and thoracic cavities. The word laparoscopy is derived from Greek words 'lapara' meaning 'the soft part of the body between the ribs and the hip, flank and loin', and 'skopein' meaning 'to look at or survey'.[4]

One of the most crucial inventions in the operative laparoscopy was by the British physicist, Harold Hopkins in the year 1952 who developed the idea of rod-lens system. Prior to this development, the conventional endoscopes were constructed with glass lenses, with long intervening air spaces. In Hopkins system, the roles of glass and air were interchanged, so that the optical medium constituted of air lenses and long glass rods.

In the previous generation, Nitze type endoscopes, the position of the lenses was maintained by 'spacer tubes', to minimize the light reflection on the inner surface.[5] This assembly resulted in the significant reduction of the viewing optic. By contrast in Hopkins glass, rods are longer and require only thin spacer tubes, clear aperture is increased. It has two problems that is light loss due to fiber mismatch at the interface of fiber optic light cable and light bundles of the telescope. The 30° angle provides a total 152° field of view compared to 76° by a 0° telescope (Figs 2.3A to D and 2.4).

Fogging is a problem encountered during surgery; warm saline is used to clean the lens with a gauze piece. Carbon dioxide (CO_2), which is used for insufflations is at lower temperature (Fig. 2.5).

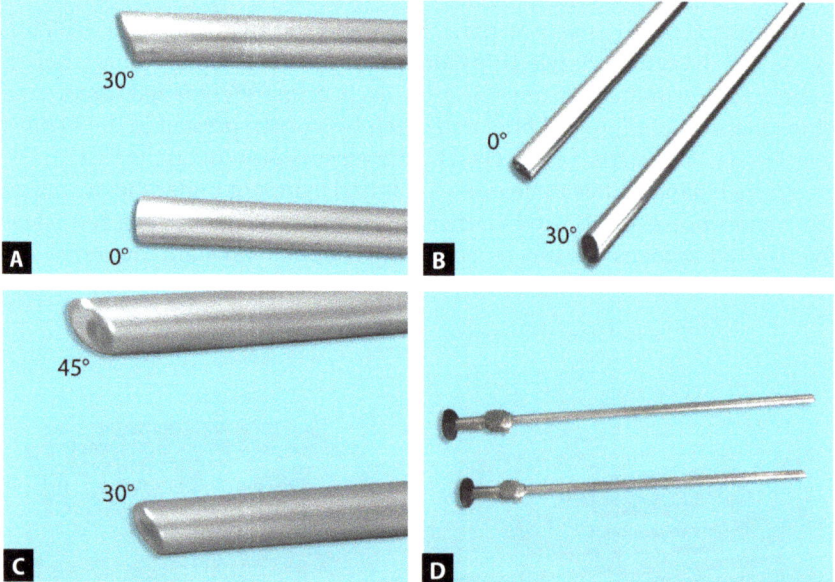

Figs 2.3A to D: Telescopes

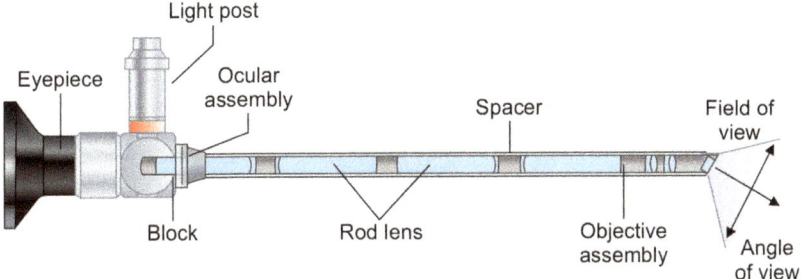

Fig. 2.4: Interiors of the telescope

Light Source

Xenon 300 watt is the commonly used light source. Xenon lamps use fused quartz as envelope with thoriated tungsten as electrodes. Fused quartz withstands high temperature and high pressure. Thorium greatly enhances the electron emission. Xenon gas inside the lamps is at very high pressure, i.e. 30 atmospheres. The smaller pointed electrode is called cathode, which emits the electrons. The larger electrode, which receives the electrons is anode. Cathode is doped with thorium and the operating temperature of the cathode is 2000°C. Atomic number of xenon is 54 (Figs 2.6 and 2.7).

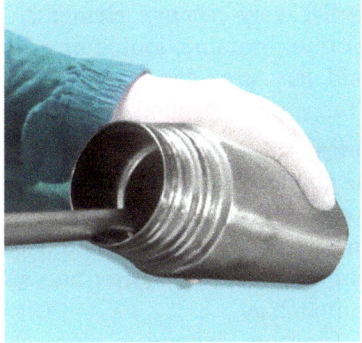

Fig. 2.5: Cleaning of the telescope tip

Incandescent Bulbs (Glowing)

Filament wire heated to a high temperature by an electric current passing through it, until it glows. Incandescent bulbs are much less efficient than most other types of electric lighting; incandescent bulbs convert less than 5% of the energy they use into visible light.[6] The hot filament is protected from oxidation by creating vacuum. In a halogen lamp, filament evaporation is prevented by a chemical process that redeposit's metal vapor onto the filament, extending its life.

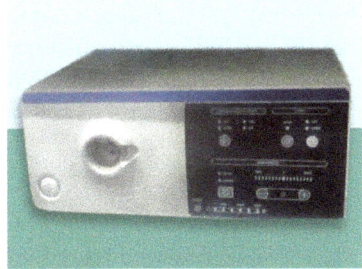

Fig. 2.6: Light source

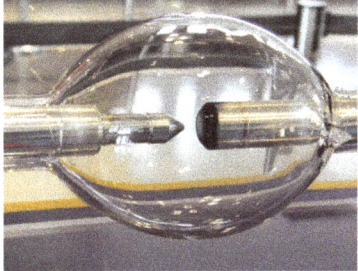

Fig. 2.7: Xenon arc light

Halogen Lamp

Halogen tungsten lamp (Fig. 2.8)
Halogen tungsten lamp is a incandescent bulb. Incandescence is glowing when heated. The true action in a halogen light bulb happens in a much smaller, tube-shaped envelope. This is made of quartz or a special glass with a higher than normal melting point. It is filled with an inert gas such as argon or xenon and a halogen, which gives the bulb its name. Halogens are five very reactive elements, fluorine, chlorine, bromine, iodine or astatine that bond very strongly with other atoms such as tungsten. The halogen usually found in a halogen bulb is iodine.

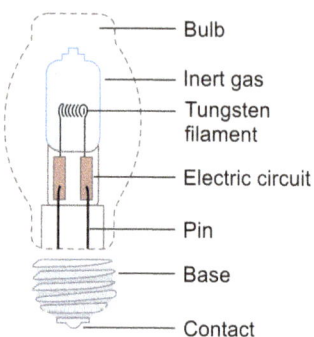

Fig. 2.8: Halogen lamp

Tungsten filament
The filament is a double coil, and heats up and glows when an electric current is passed through it. Heating up and glowing is simply a function how fast the tungsten atoms vibrate. A bulb with a longer filament has a higher wattage than a bulb with a shorter one, simply because of the amount of atoms the filament has.

Tungsten is the usual element for light bulb filaments, because it is easy to draw into an extremely thin wire and has a very high melting point of over 6,000°F. Even a halogen light does not get that hot—it gets to about 5,400°F at its hottest—so the tungsten does not melt. Still, the heat in even a regular incandescent bulb causes the tungsten to evaporate and blacken inside of the bulb, but in a halogen light bulb the tungsten reacts with the halogen and is redeposited on the filament coil, which helps to extend the life of the bulb.

Electric circuit
The electric circuit is connected to the filament and allows an electric current to pass through it, to the point where it glows. The current travels up from one of the wires, across the filament and then travels down the wire on the other side.

Pin
The pin anchors the electrical wires into the stem of the bulb and helps to bring the current up and down the electrical circuit.

Base
Halogen light bulbs can come with bases that can screw into the socket of a light fixture. The screw base is usually insulated with vitrite.

Contact
When it touches the contact of the light fixture, the contact of the halogen light bulb allows electricity to flow through the electrical circuit and cause the filament to glow.

Total Internal Reflection

Total internal reflection is the operating principle of the optical fibers, which are used in endoscopes (Figs 2.9 and 2.10).

If the refractive index is lower on the other side of the boundary and the incident angle is greater than the critical angle, the wave cannot pass through and is entirely reflected.

When a wave crosses a boundary between materials with different kinds of refractive indices, the wave will be partially refracted at the boundary surface and partially reflected. However, if the angle of incidence is greater (i.e. the direction of propagation or ray is closer to being parallel to the boundary) than the critical angle—the angle of incidence at which light is refracted such that it travels along the boundary, then the wave will not cross the boundary and instead be totally reflected back internally. This can only occur where the wave travels from a medium with a higher refractive index (n_1) to one with a lower refractive index (n_2). For example, it will occur with light when passing from glass to air, but not when passing from air to glass.

When light traveling in an optically dense medium hits a boundary at a steep angle (larger than the critical angle for the boundary), the light is completely reflected. This is called total internal reflection. This effect is used in optical fibers to confine light in the core. Light travels through the fiber core, bouncing back and forth off the boundary between the core and cladding.

Optical fibers[7] typically include a transparent core surrounded by a transparent cladding material with a lower index of refraction. Light is kept in the core by total internal reflection (Fig. 2.11).

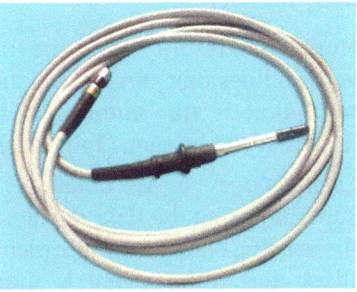

Fig. 2.9: Total internal reflection

Monitors

Television systems differ according to the countries. The USA uses the NTSC system and in European countries PAL is used.

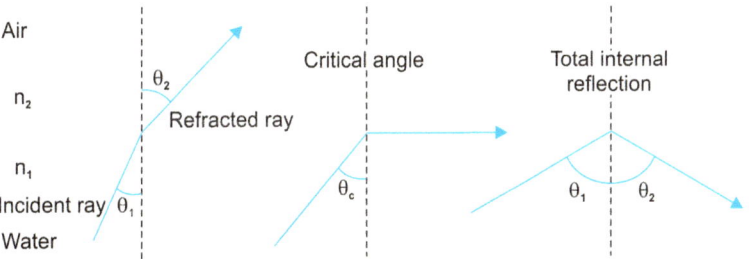

Fig. 2.10: Principle of optics: Total internal reflection

Monitor Specifications (Requirements)

Horizontal resolution is the number of vertical lines that can be seen and vertical resolution is the number of horizontal lines that can be seen (Table 2.1).[8]

Color image: It is obtained by superimposing the data of color on the existing black and white picture. Black and white signal is monochromatic, which is combined with the composite color signal.[9]

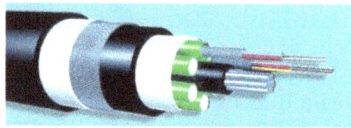

Fig. 2.11: Optical fiber cable

Table 2.1: Monitor specifications

System	PAL*	NTSC†
Number of lines (visible lines)	625 (575)	525 (486)
Cycles per second	50	60
Frames per second	25	30

*PAL, phase alternating line; †NTSC, National Television System Committee.

REFERENCES

1. Bruce V Macfadyen Jr. Laparoscopic Surgery of the Abdomen, Laparoscopic Instrumentation, New York: Springer-Verlag; 2004. pp. 335-51.
2. C Palanivelu. Art of Laparoscopic Surgery Textbook and Atlas. New Delhi: Jaypee Brothers Medical Publishers (P) Ltd; 2005. pp. 11-34.
3. RK Mishra, Textbook of Practical laparoscopic Surgery, laparoscopic imaging systems, 3rd edition. New Delhi: Jaypee Brothers Medical Publishers (P) Ltd; 2013. pp. 9-29.
4. Berkelium BM. Organoscopy:cystoscopy of the abdominal cavity. Ann Surg. 1911;53(6):764-7.
5. Semm K. Endoscopic intraabdominal surgery, 2nd edition. Kiel; 1984.
6. "The Nature of Light". Archived from the original on 2012-07-24. Retrieved 2007-11-05.
7. Knyrim K, Scidilitz H, Vakil N, et al. Perspectives in "electronic endoscopy." Past present and future of fibers and CCDS in medical endoscopes. Endoscopy. 1990; (Suppl 1):2-8.
8. Hanna GB, Cusheri A. Influence of two-dimensional and three-dimensional imaging on endoscopic bowel suturing. World J Surgery. 2000;24(4):444-9.
9. Berci G Davids J, et al. Endoscopy and television. Br Med J. 1962;1(5229):1610-3.

CHAPTER 3

Instruments

LAPAROSCOPIC HAND INSTRUMENTS

The laparoscopic instruments range in size from 18 to 45 cm (Fig. 3.1). The instruments that are routinely used are 33 cm in size and 45 cm instruments are used in obese individuals. The laparoscopic hand instruments can be dismantled into three parts, i.e. inner effector, outer sheath and hand grip (Figs 3.2 to 3.4). For better ergonomics half of the instrument should be within the abdomen and half should be outside.

Some handles are provided with locking mechanism, the locking mechanism prevents the fatigability of the surgeon's hand. There are two types of ratchet. Usually, the handles are provided with monopolar electrosurgical lead for the cable to be connected (Fig. 3.5). They have a rotator mechanism for rotation of the tip (Fig. 3.6).

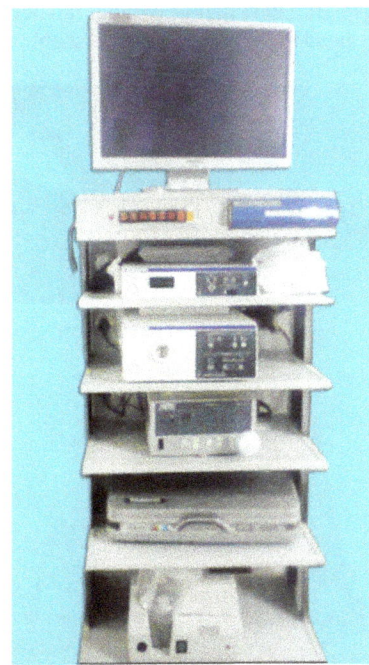

Fig. 3.1: Laparoscopy unit

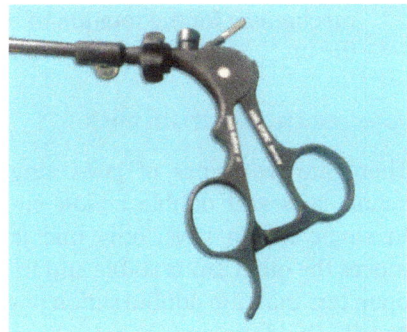

Fig. 3.2: Hand grip with ratchet

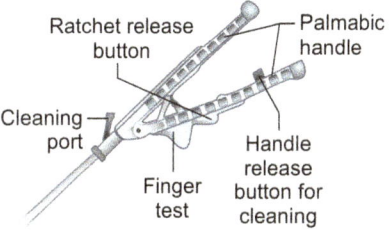

Fig. 3.3: Mechanism of hand grip

Features of Ideal Instrument[2]

1. The instrument should be simple with minimum hinges and bolts (Figs 3.7 and 3.8).
2. The jaws of the hand instrument should be atraumatic.
3. The instruments should be easy to dismantle (Fig. 3.9) and reassemble.
4. The commercially available counterparts should be interchangeable.
5. Cleaning and sterilization should be easy.
6. The outer sheath should be replaced easily.
7. Checking the function of the instrument should be easy.
8. The various parts of the hand instrument should be easily available in the market, so that only the defective part needs to be replaced.
9. They should have an electrosurgical lead.
10. They should have a rotator mechanism for the rotation of the tip.

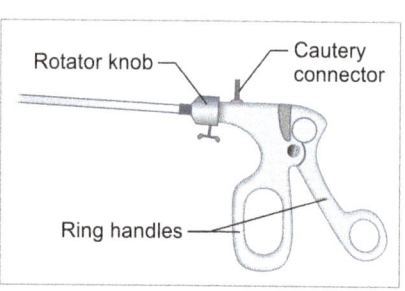

Fig. 3.4: Hand grip

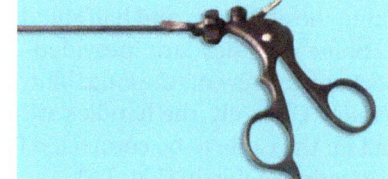

Fig. 3.5: Ring handle without ratchet (lead for the cautery cord is seen)

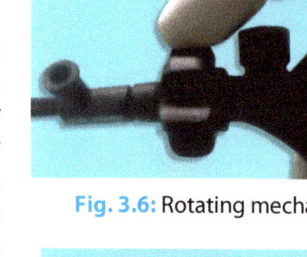

Fig. 3.6: Rotating mechanism

Jaws of the Instruments

There are two types of jaws, single action jaws and double action jaws. In single action jaws, only one jaw moves the other jaw is stable and they open less than the double action jaws. Needle holders and some scissors are examples of single action jaws. In double action jaws both the jaws move as in graspers (Fig. 3.10) and dissecting forceps.

Scissors

Application of cautery to the scissors reduces the sharpness of the instrument therefore this should be avoided.[3]

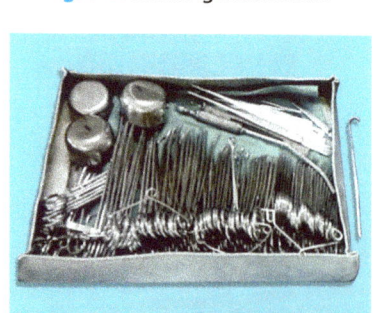

Fig. 3.7: Instrument tray

Types (Figs 3.11 and 3.12)

1. Straight scissors.
2. Curved scissors.
3. *Serrated scissors:* The advantage with the serrated scissors is that they do not allow the tissue to slip.
4. *Hook scissors:* Both the jaws are curved and sharp, there are no chances of sliping. Other scissors cut from proximal to distal, but hook scissors cut in both direction.
5. *Microtip scissors:* They are fine scissors, may be straight or curved, mainly used for cutting the common bile duct for exploration or the cystic duct for performing the intraoperative cholangiography.

Spatula

Metal instrument used in laparoscopic procedures such as dissection or holding the parts (Figs 3.13 and 3.14).

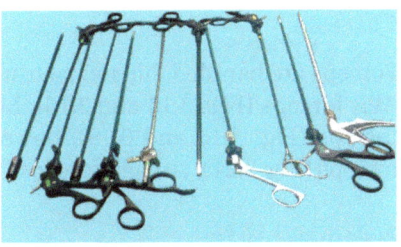

Fig. 3.8: Laparoscopic instruments

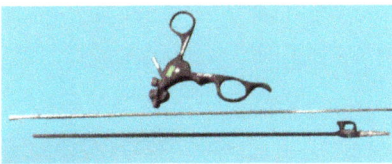

Fig. 3.9: Dismantled laparoscopic hand instrument: Hand grip, inner effector and outer sheath.

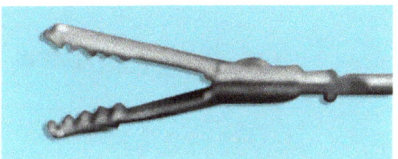

Fig. 3.10: Grasper

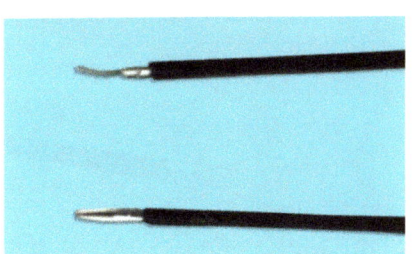

Fig. 3.11: Curved and straight scissor

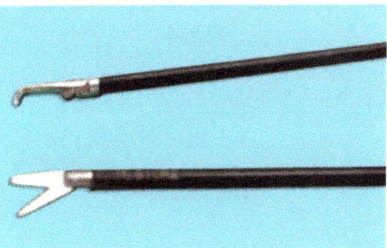

Fig. 3.12: Right-angled forceps, scissor

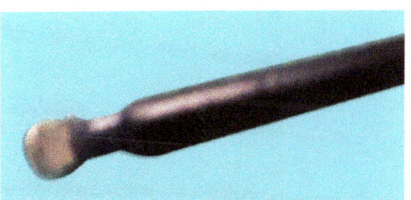

Fig. 3.13: Spatula

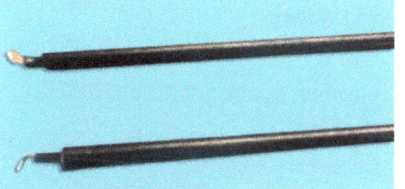

Fig. 3.14: Spatula and hook used to dissect the gallbladder from its bed

Forceps

Forceps are handled, hinged instruments used for grasping and holding, e.g. Allis forceps (Figs 3.15 and 3.16), Maryland forceps (Fig. 3.17), saw-toothed forceps (Figs 3.18 and 3.19), bowel holding forceps (Fig. 3.20), Babcock's forceps (Fig. 3.21), straight forceps (Figs 3.22 and 3.23), etc.

Needle Holder

Needle holders (Fig. 3.24) are strong and heavy. They have single moving jaw and tapering tip. The tip of the instrument can be either straight or curved.

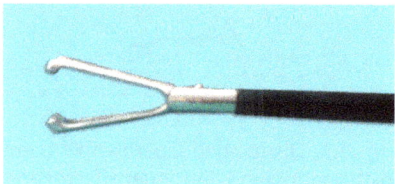

Fig. 3.15: Allis forceps (photograph)

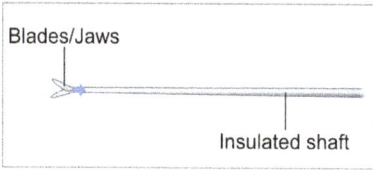

Fig. 3.16: Allis forceps (diagrammatic representation)

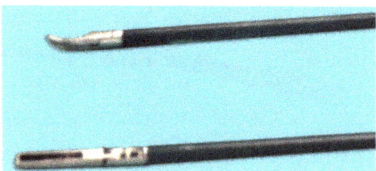

Fig. 3.17: Maryland forceps and Allis forceps

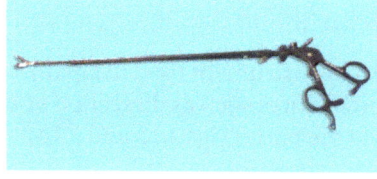

Fig. 3.18: Saw-toothed forceps

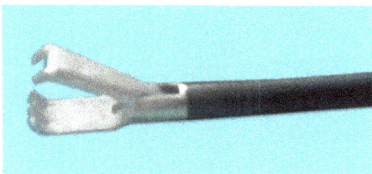

Fig. 3.19: Saw-toothed forceps

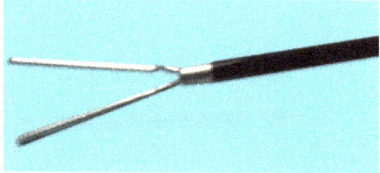

Fig. 3.20: Bowel holding forceps

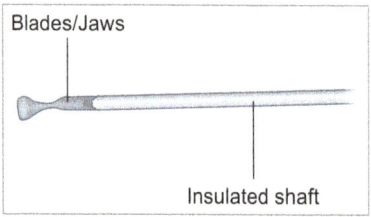

Fig. 3.21: Babcock's forceps

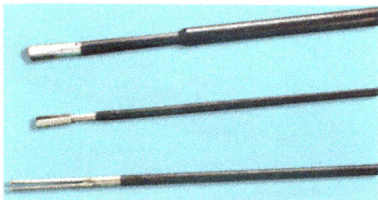

Fig. 3.22: Saw-toothed forceps, straight forceps and bowel holding forceps

Instruments **17**

Coaxial handles (Fig. 3.25) are preferred to pistol handle. The jaws are serrated and one of the jaw may be concave or flat. In line grip, needle holders are better ergonomic than the pitol grip needle holder.

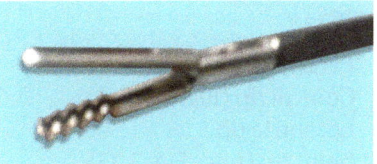

Fig. 3.23: Straight forceps with transverse ridges

Insulation

The insulation is made up of plastic. Care should be taken, while cleaning the instruments as any breach in the insulation will cause leak during electrosurgery.

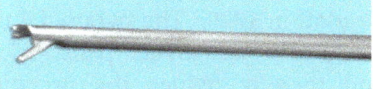

Fig. 3.24: Needle holder

Trocar

The word trocar is usually used for the entire assembly, but actually it is only the tip of stylet, which is introduced through the cannula (Fig. 3.26) . Trocar (Fig. 3.27) refers to the sharp end of the assembly, which penetrates the abdominal wall. Trocars are available in disposable (Figs 3.28 to 3.30) and reusable forms. They range in size from 3 to 30 mm (Fig. 3.31), but the commonly used once are 5 and 10 mm (Figs 3.32 and 3.33). Metal trocars have different types of tips.

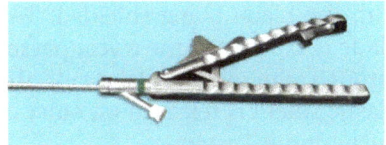

Fig. 3.25: Needle holder handle (coaxial grip)

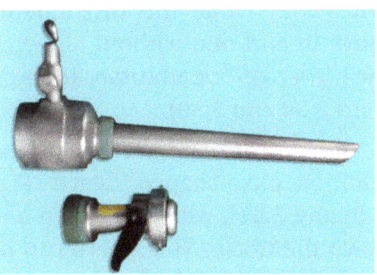

Fig. 3.26: Outer sheath of trocar and valve

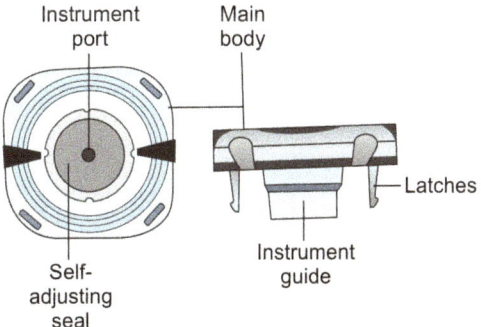

Fig. 3.27: Description of trocar

Types

- Pyramidal tip (Fig. 3.34)
- Conical tip (Fig. 3.35)
- Eccentric tip
- Blunt tip (refer Fig. 3.35).

Peritoneal access was facilitated by the introduction of pyramidal shaped sharp tipped trocars by Orndoff in 1920.[1] The pyramidal tip trocars penetrate by sharp dissection and thereby reduce the pressure required to transverse the abdominal wall. Some trocars are designed with the blade being shielded. The blade is exposed as the trocar passes through the abdominal wall, the plastic shield is released on entry of the peritoneal cavity.

Cannulas do have valves (Fig. 3.36), which provide air seal (Fig. 3.37) while the instruments move in and out, without allowing the loss of pneumoperitoneum (Figs 3.38 and 3.39).

Hasson trocar: The trocar has an addition olive-shaped sleeve (Figs 3.40 and 3.41), which slides up and down the trocar. This sleeve can be fixed to the abdominal wall by taking stitches in the fascia. The sharp obturator is replaced by a blunt one in order to reduce the injury to the organs. The sleeve has two transverse ridges that are used to fix the conical sleeve to the fascia with the help of suture material.

Valve

Trumpet valve: The outer knob has to be pressed completely for insertion and removal of the instruments.

Flap valve: They are spring loaded. The valves have to be dismantled

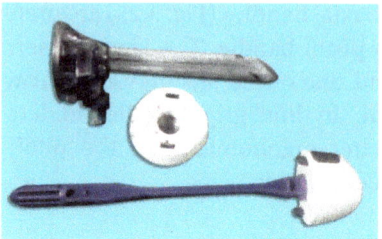

Fig. 3.28: 12 mm disposable trocar dismantaled, cap, sheath and obturator

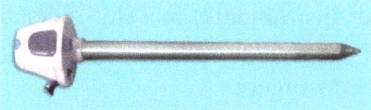

Fig. 3.29: Optical view of disposable trocar were scope can be introduced to view the puncture

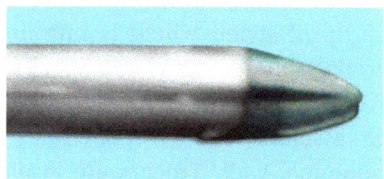

Fig. 3.30: 12 mm disposable trocar tip (optiview)

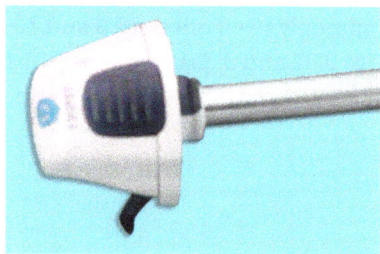

Fig. 3.31: 12 mm trocar

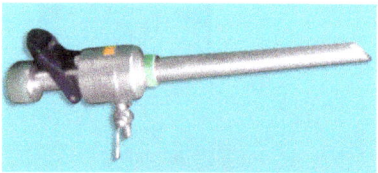

Fig. 3.32: 10 mm cannula with valve and gas inlet

Instruments **19**

and cleaned thoroughly in order to remove the blood clots lodged in them (Fig. 3.42).

Reducer

Reducer are the instruments (Figs 3.43 to 3.45) used to convert the 10 mm cannulas to 5 mm. It will help in maintaining the pneumoperitoneum, whenever there is change in the instruments from larger to smaller diameter.

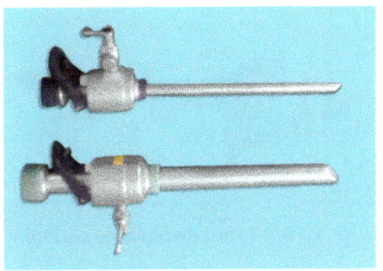

Fig. 3.33: 5 and 10 mm cannula

Clip Applicators (Figs. 3.46 to 3.52)

Disposable clip appliers come with preloaded clips usually 20 in number, the advantage is every time clip is applied there is no necessity to remove the clip applier for reloading, this will save time. The disadvantage is they are costly. Absorbable clips are sometimes used. The jaws of the clip applicator should be at right angles to the structure applied. Both the jaws should be seen before application. Clips are made up of titanium and are inert. When applied to the cystic duct two clips are towards the CBD and one towards the specimen.

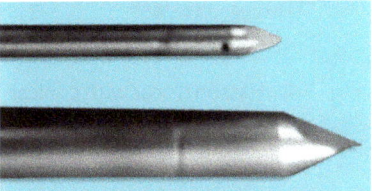

Fig. 3.34: Pyramidal tip obturator

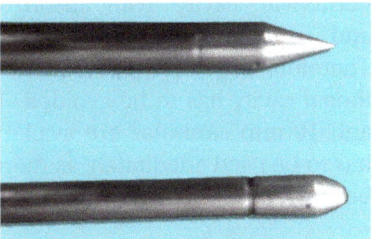

Fig. 3.35: Conical tip and blunt tip.

The distance between the clip legs is 4.5 mm before application. Titanium clips do not interfere with either computed tomography (CT) or magnetic resonance imaging (MRI).

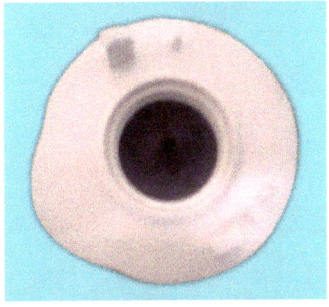

Fig. 3.36: Valve in the cap

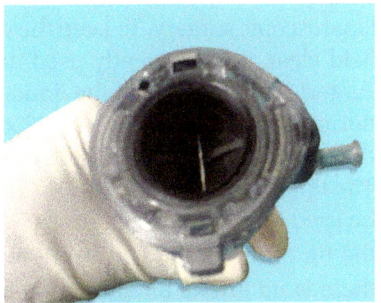

Fig. 3.37: Self-adjusting seal of the outer sheath

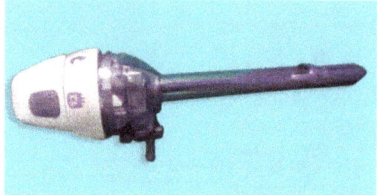

Fig. 3.38: 12 mm disposable cannula

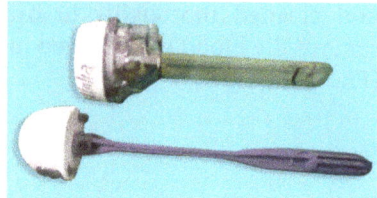

Fig. 3.39: Cannula and obturator

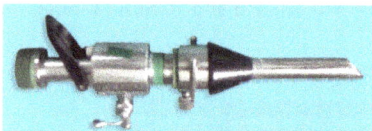

Fig. 3.40: Hasson trocar with conical sleeve

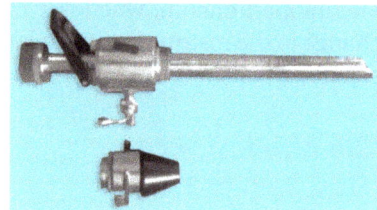

Fig. 3.41: Cannula and Hasson sleeve

Suction Irrigation System

Even a small quantity of blood in the peritoneal cavity will absorb light and cause insufficient illumination. Therefore, blood collection in the peritoneal cavity has to be avoided. The 5 and 10 mm cannulas are available. It has to be used adequately as there will be sudden loss of pneumoperitoneum.

Suction and Irrigation

The irrigation apparatus (Figs 3.53 and 3.54) increase the pressure within reservoir, which pushes the fluid through the tubes. It is used for flushing the abdominal cavity and cleaning during laparoscopic surgery. To keep the visual field clear, it is frequently used during surgery. Vision is one of the limitations during laparoscopic surgery, blood in the peritoneal cavity will absorb the light. The tip of the probe (Fig. 3.55) can also be used for blunt dissection. As long as the tip of the probe is within the fluid there is no loss of pneumoperitoneum once the fluid gets over, there will be drastic loss of pneumoperitoneum.

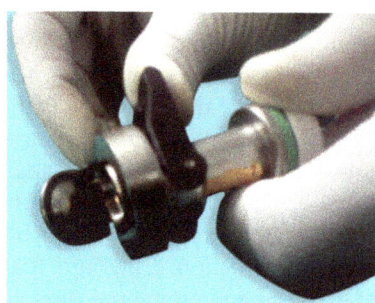

Fig. 3.42: Flap valve

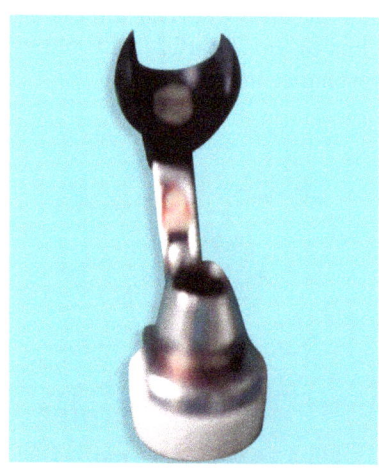

Fig. 3.43: Reducer

Instruments

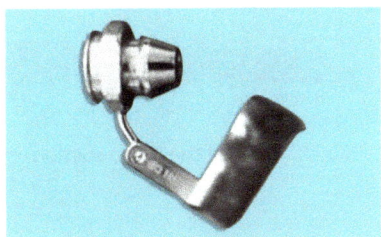

Fig. 3.44: 10–5 mm reducer

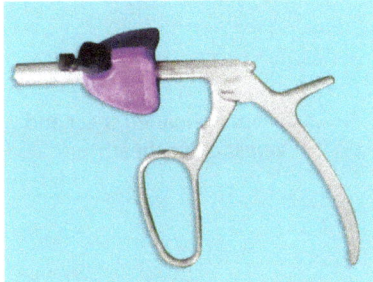

Fig. 3.46: Handle of clip applicator

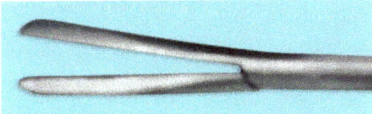

Fig. 3.48: Jaws of clip applicator

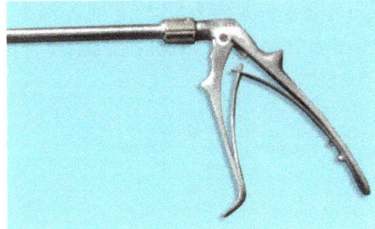

Fig. 3.50: Clip applicator handle

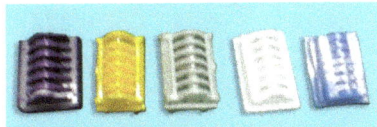

Fig. 3.52: Clips: Violet (ligaclip, hemlock); yellow (11 mm); green (9 mm); white (7 mm); blue (5 mm).

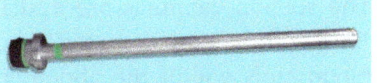

Fig. 3.45: Sleeve reducer-1

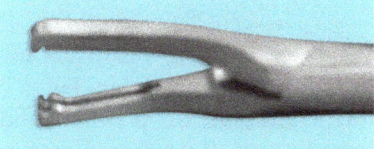

Fig. 3.47: Jaws of clip applicator

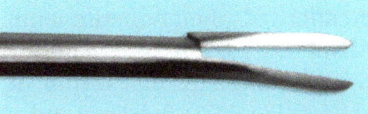

Fig. 3.49: Different clip applicator

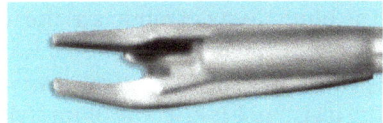

Fig. 3.51: Clip applicator jaws

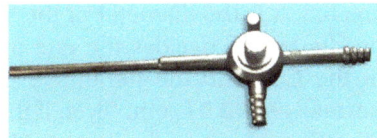

Fig. 3.53: Handle of suction

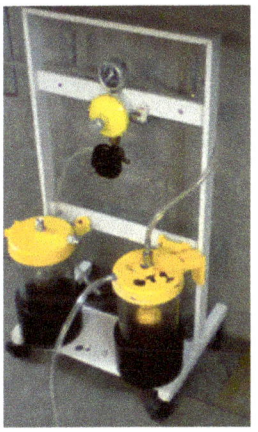

Fig. 3.54: Suction apparatus

The suction cannulas are available in 10 mm and 5 mm diameter, if there are blood clots within the abdomen then 10 mm cannula can be used.

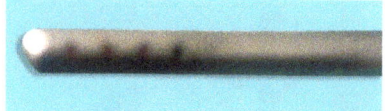

Fig. 3.55: Tip of the 5 mm suction nozzle

Veress Needle

Veress needle (Fig. 3.56) was invented by Hungarian physician Janos Veress for aspiration of pleural fluid and introduction of pneumothorax in pulmonary tuberculosis in the year 1938. But today it is extensively used for the creation of pneumoperitoneum.[9] It is about 10–15 cm in length, with an outside diameter of 1.8 mm. It has a sheath (Fig. 3.57), the distal end of which is beveled. The inner stylet is blunt tipped and spring loaded (Fig. 3.58). The blunt tip stylet retracts as the needle passes through the abdominal wall, but springs into the peritoneal cavity once the resistance is lost. The blunt stylet has a lateral hole in the distal end through which the pneumoperitoneum can be created. It is the diameter of the Veress needle, which decides the rate of flow of the CO_2 into the peritoneal cavity, normally it is 2.5 L/min. Even if the rate of setting is kept on the higher side, it is limited by the diameter and the lateral hole in the stylet.

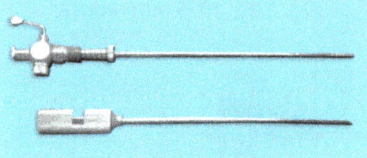

Fig. 3.57: Spring-loaded stylet and Veress outer sheath

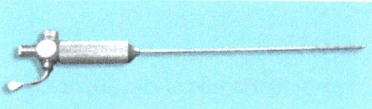

Fig. 3.56: Veress needle

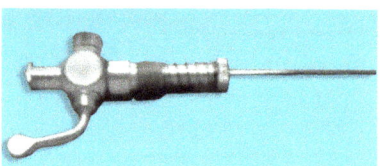

Fig. 3.58: Spring-loaded stylet

Tackers

Tackers are mechanical fixation devices used in surgery. They come in different configurations. Some are in the form of coils that are screwed in the tissue. While applying the tackers, counter pressure has to be applied for the tacker to fix properly.

Endoanchor (Fig. 3.59) from ethicon endosurgery has two lateral extensions, proximal and distal.

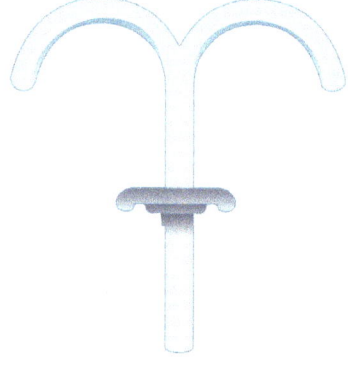

Fig. 3.59: Anchor-shaped secure strap

Secure strap has a U-shaped configuration (Fig. 3.60) with lateral projections from the limbs of U. Where the limbs of U will go through the pores in the mesh to fix it to the abdominal wall.

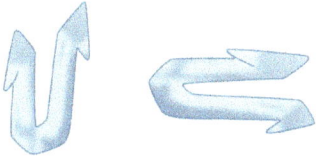

Fig. 3.60: U-shaped secure strap

■ REFERENCES

1. Harrell AG, Heniford BT. Minimally invasive abdominal surgery: lux et veritas past, present, and future. Am J Surg. 2005;190(2):239-43.
2. Matern U, Waller P. Instruments for minimally invasive surgery: principles of ergonomic handles. Surg Endosc. 1999;13(2):174-82.
3. C Palanivelu. Art of Laparoscopic Surgery Textbook and Atlas. vol 1. Instrumentation and imaging systems in laparoscopy. New Delhi; Jaypee Brothers Medical Publishers (P) Ltd; 2007. pp. 11-35.

CHAPTER 4

Pneumoperitoneum

Pneumoperitoneum was maintained by syringe injections until Goetze described manual insufflators in 1921. A Swiss gynecologist Richard Zollikofer popularized carbon dioxide (CO_2) insufflation in 1924 as it was absorbed faster and noninflammable. Stone of the United States dramatically reduced the leakage of gas through the trocars with rubber gasket.[1]

Fervers, a gynecologist did laparoscopic therapeutic adhesiolysis in the year 1933, he used oxygen for pneumoperitoneum and experienced 'great concern' at the audible explosion and flashes of light produced by combustion of oxygen by cautery. He recommended changing to CO_2 for creation of pneumoperitoneum.[2] Kurt Semm developed the insufflators in the year 1960.[3] Palmer stressed the importance of monitoring the intra-abdominal pressure.

INSUFFLATORS

The intra-abdominal pressure should be maintained at 12–14 mm of Hg in order to avoid complications of gas embolism and decreased venous return due to pressure on inferior vena cava.[4]

Modern insufflators (Figs 4.1 and 4.2) infuse gas in the peritoneum at a predetermined rate by electronic mechanism. They monitor the intra-abdominal pressure constantly, the flow stops on reaching the set pressure and resumes when the pressure decreases due to leakage or suction. The first column indicates the set intraperitoneal pressure, this is done by the surgeon. The second column indicates the rate of flow, which is also set flow. The third indicator shows the amount of gas utilized (in liters).

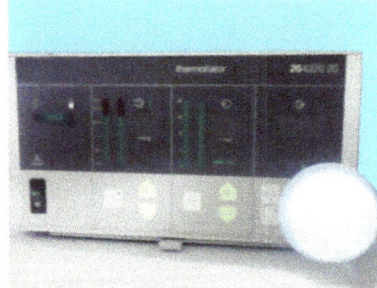

Fig. 4.1: Insufflator

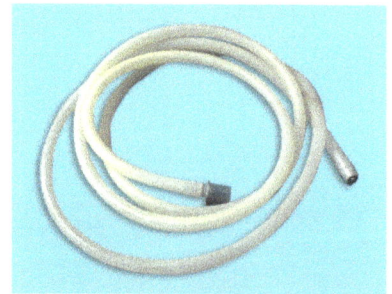

Fig. 4.2: Insufflating tube

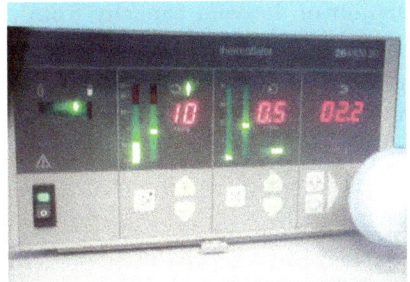 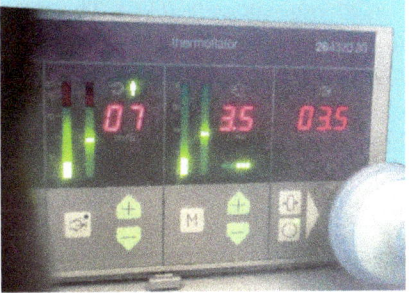

Fig. 4.3: Insufflator with three columns—the first showing set intra-abdominal pressure (mm Hg), second showing rate of flow (L/min), third showing volume of gas utilized in liters

Fig. 4.4: Insufflator with three readings—the first showing set intra-abdominal pressure (mm Hg), second showing rate of flow (L/min), third showing volume of gas utilized in liters

In Figure 4.3 (pneumoperitoneum is in progress) the first column shows the intraperitoneal pressure, the second column (0.5 L/min) shows the rate flow through the Veress needle and third column indicates the volume of gas utilized (2.2 liters). In Figure 4.4, pneumoperitoneum is in progress.

TERMINOLOGIES

Total lung capacity (TLC): The volume in the lungs at maximal inflation, the sum of vital capacity (VC) and residual volume (RV).

Tidal volume (V_T): That volume of air moved into or out of the lungs during quiet breathing (VT indicates a subdivision of the lung; when tidal volume is precisely measured, as in gas exchange calculation, the symbol V_T or VT is used).

Residual volume (RV): The volume of air remaining in the lungs after a maximal exhalation.

Expiratory reserve volume (ERV): The maximal volume of air that can be exhaled from the end-expiratory position.

Inspiratory reserve volume (IRV): The maximal volume that can be inhaled from the end-inspiratory level.

Inspiratory capacity (IC): The sum of IRV and V_T.

Inspiratory vital capacity (IVC): The maximum volume of air inhaled from the point of maximum expiration.

Vital capacity (VC): The volume of air breathed out after the deepest inhalation.

Functional residual capacity (FRC): The volume in the lungs at the end-expiratory position.

Residual volume (RV): It is expressed as percent of TLC (RV/TLC%).

Alveolar gas volume (AV): Actual volume of the lung including the volume of the conducting airway.

Forced vital capacity (FVC): The determination of the vital capacity from a maximally forced expiratory effort.

Forced expiratory volume (time) (FEV_t): A generic term indicating the volume of air exhaled under forced conditions in the first t seconds. Volume that has been exhaled at the end of the first second of forced expiration (FEV_1).

Forced expiratory flow (FEFx): It is related to some portion of the FVC curve; modifiers refer to amount of FVC already exhaled.

FEFmax: The maximum instantaneous flow achieved during an FVC maneuver.

Forced inspiratory flow (FIF): Specific measurement of the forced inspiratory curve is denoted by nomenclature analogous to that for the forced expiratory curve. For example, maximum inspiratory flow is denoted as FIFmax. Unless otherwise specified, volume qualifiers indicate the volume inspired from RV at the point of measurement.

Peak expiratory flow (PEF): The highest forced expiratory flow is measured with a peak flow meter.

Maximal voluntary ventilation (MVV): Volume of air expired in a specified period during repetitive maximal effort.

PNEUMOPERITONEUM INSUFFLATION

Physiological Changes (Fig. 4.5)

Respiratory Changes

Carbon dioxide is the commonly used insufflating agent in laparoscopy. This is due to its easy availability, relatively inexpensive, noncombustible and high

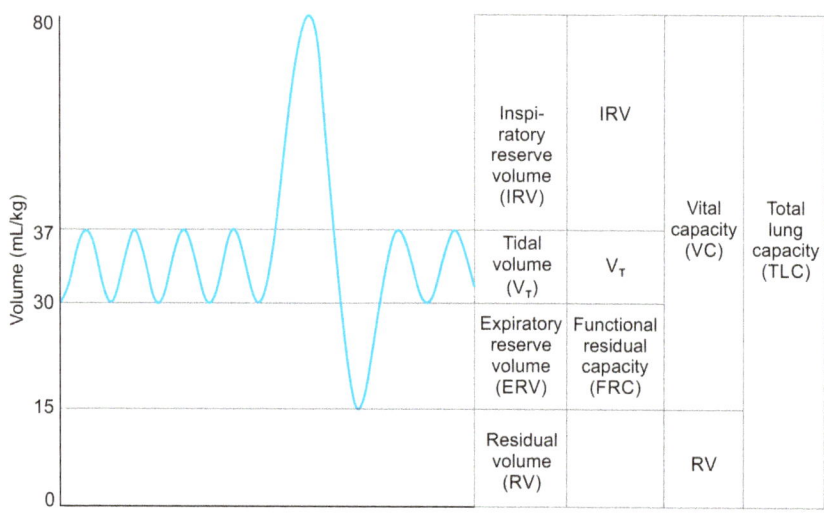

Fig. 4.5: Physiological changes in laparoscopy

solubility minimizing the gas embolism. It is absorbed by the peritoneal cavity and carried by the systemic and portal veins and is excreted by the lungs. Carbon dioxide production (VCO_2) increases gradually and reaches a plateau after 20 minutes at 125% of the baseline.[5] The diaphragm is shifted upwards resulting in reduction of lung volume and FRC. Airway resistance is increased. The anesthetist uses high airway pressure to overcome the resistance.

Alveolar gas exchange requires adequate ventilation and perfusion (V/Q). Normally, they are fairly well matched, ratio of 4 L/min of ventilation to 5 L/min of perfusion (blood flow). There is ventilation and perfusion mismatch in laparoscopy.

Cardiovascular Changes

Cardiac output decreases with pneumoperitoneum (as much as 50%). It depends on three factors, i.e. myocardial function, preload and afterload.

The venous return from the lower part of the body is reduced, but the CVP is raised. This is because of rise in intrathoracic pressure. The venous return is reduced, because of the pressure effect on the inferior vena cava.[3]

Blood pressure increases due to raised systemic vascular resistance. The blood pressure takes some time to come to normal after exsufflation. This is explained on the basis of humoral factors such as catecholamines, rennin, vasopressin. Among them vasopressin is important. Raised IAP causes reduced blood flow to the intra-abdominal organs. splanchnic, mesenteric and intestinal mucosal blood flow are decreased. The intestinal ischemia gives rise to decreased intestinal mucosal pH. Renal blood flow is reduced along with decreased glomerular filtrate and urine output.

Patient Position

Supine position causes the patient's diaphragm to elevate and results in 20% reduction of functional residual capacity, pneumoperitoneum also reduces FRC.[1] Head down position increases the venous return, central venous pressure and the stroke volume, but the arterial pressure does not change significantly because of the vasodilatation and bradycardia.[2]

Trendelenburg position also increases the intracranial pressure and intraocular pressure, hence should be avoided in increased ICP and acute glaucoma. Reverse Trendelenburg position decreases venous return and cardiac output. But it increases the respiratory function, therefore it is the preferred position as far as respiratory system is concerned. Lithotomy position will lead to 40–45% loss of FRC, this loss increases with Trendelenburg position. Lateral positions also reduce the FRC.

Ideal Insufflating Agents

1. Insufflating agent should be inert, colorless and noninflammable.
2. High solubility in the blood.
3. It should be cheap, easily available and nontoxic.

The various insufflating agents available are air, carbondioxide, nitrous oxide, helium, argon. Nitrogen has been proposed as an insufflating agent.[6]

Air

Initially, air was used for creation of pneumoperitoneum. The main disadvantage is air embolism, as 1 mL of air in the coronary circulation is sufficient to cause death.[4]

Carbon Dioxide

Carbon dioxide is almost universally used as the insufflating agent to create laparoscopic pneumoperitoneum. It is cheap, noncombustible and colorless. It is easily excreted by lungs during normal respiration, but the very characteristic feature of CO_2 is it is highly soluble in water thereby reducing the chances of embolism drastically.[1]

Metabolic effects of CO_2

Carbon dioxide is absorbed by the peritoneal surface in addition to the CO_2 being produced by the normal metabolic processes of the body, leading to systemic acidosis and hypercapnia. It can be stored in the bone skeletal muscles and other tissues.[5] There is direct correlation between the amount of CO_2 utilized and increase in the partial pressure of CO_2. Cardiorespiratory effects of pneumoperitoneum give rise to decreased return of blood from the lower extremities and the pelvis. There is also significant alteration in the CVP, cardiac output, cardiac rhythm, splanchnic and mesenteric blood flow.[7]

Acting on the cardia directly it causes bradycardia, decreased cardiac contractility. On the other hand due to sympathetic stimulation there is tachycardia, increased systolic and diastolic blood pressure, and peripheral vasoconstriction. Sustained high levels may lead to arrhythmias and death.[4]

Immunological effects

Peritoneal macrophages play an important role in the primary inflammatory response to infection and cancer. The scavenging action of these macrophages is mediated in part by the production of inflammatory cytokines such TNF-α. CO_2 insufflation impairs the peritoneal macrophages to produce TNF-α.[8]

Helium

Helium is inert and colorless gas and does not support combustion (noninflammable). Acidosis and hypercarbia as seen with CO_2 insufflation are not seen with helium.[9,10] The drawback is 50 times less soluble than CO_2 in the blood thus increasing the chances of gas embolism.[11] Subcutaneous emphysema that occurs with helium stays longer.[12]

Argon

Like helium argon is inert, noninflammable, inexpensive and easily available.[9,12,13] The disadvantage is it is relatively insoluble in blood, therefore it may carry the same gas embolism potential as helium.[7]

Nitrous Oxide

Nitrogen is the gaseous element found freely in the air. Nitrous oxide was the preferred gas for pneumoperitoneum in the 1970s and 80s.[14] But concerns about its combustibility and cases of explosion in the operation theater during female sterilization using electrocautery led to decline in its usage.[15]

■ REFERENCES

1. Harrell AG. Minimally invasive abdominal surgery: Lux, et al. Veritas past, present and future. Am J Surg. 2005;190(2):239-43.
2. Gorden A. The history and development of endoscopic surgery. Endoscopic surgery for gynaecologists. Saunders; 1993. pp. 3-7.
3. Lau WY, et al. History of endoscopic and laparoscopic surgery. World J Surg. 1997;21:444-53.
4. C Palanivelu. Art of Laparoscopic Surgery: Textbook and Atlas. vol 1. 2007. pp. 19-20.
5. Naude GP, et al. Helium insufflations in laparoscopic surgery. Endosc Surg Allied Technol. 1995;3(4):183-6.
6. Aneman A, et al. Intestinal perfusion during pneumoperitoneum with CO_2, nitrogen and nitrous oxide during laparoscopic surgery. Eur J Surg. 2000;166(1): 70-6.
7. Martin IG, et al. Gasless laparoscopy. JR Coll Surg Edinb. 1996;41(2):72-4.
8. Neuhaus SJ, et al. The influence of different gases on the intraperitoneal immunity in the tumor bearing rats. World J Surg. 2000;24:1227-31.
9. Steuer K. Pneumoperitoneum—physiology and nursing interventions. AORN J. 1998;68(3):412-25.
10. Bongard FS, et al. Using helium for insufflations during laparoscopy. JAMA. 1991;266(22):3131.
11. Wolf Jr, et al. Gas embolism; helium is more lethal than CO_2. J Laparoendoscopic Surg. 1994;4(3):173-7.
12. Macmohan, et al. Helium pneumoperitoneum for laparoscopic cholecystectomy: ventilator and blood gas changes. Br J Surg. 1994;81(7):1033-6.
13. Neuhaus SJ, et al. Helium and other alternative insufflations gases for laparoscopy. Surg Endoscopy. 2001;15:553-60.
14. Eisenhauer DM, et al. Hemodynamic effects of argon pneumoperitoneum. Surg Endoscopy. 1994;8(4):315-20.
15. Aitola P, et al. Comparsion of nitrous oxide and carbon dioxide pneumoperitoneum during laparoscopic cholecystectomy with sp reference to postoperative pain. Surg Laparoendosc. 1998;8:140-4.

CHAPTER 5

Peritoneal Access

ANATOMY OF ANTERIOR ABDOMINAL WALL

There are three large flat muscles (external oblique, internal oblique and transverse abdominis muscles) laterally and one long vertical segmental muscle (rectus abdominis) medially, on each side. The superior and inferior epigastric arteries supply blood to the rectus abdominis muscle. Umbilicus is a scar in the anterior abdominal wall. At this level, the skin fascia and the peritoneum are fused and there is minimal fat.

METHODS OF PERITONEAL ACCESS

The four basic techniques used for creation of pneumoperitoneum are:
1. Veress needle technique.
2. Direct trocar insertion.
3. Optical trocar insertion.
4. Open technique (Hasson).

The first two are blind and the last two are performed under vision.

Closed Technique

Veress needle was invented by Hungarian physician Janos Veress for aspiration of pleural fluid and introduction of pneumothorax in pulmonary tuberculosis in the year 1938 (Figs 5.1 and 5.2). But today it is extensively used for the creation of pneumoperitoneum.[1] It is about 10–15 cm in length, with an outside diameter of 1.8 mm. It has a sheath, the distal end of which is beveled.[2] The inner stylet is blunt tipped and spring loaded. The blunt tip stylet retracts as the needle passes through the abdominal wall, but springs into the peritoneal cavity once the resistance is lost. The blunt stylet has a lateral hole in the distal end through which the pneumoperitoneum can be created. It is the diameter of the Veress needle, which decides the rate of flow of CO_2 into the peritoneal cavity. Normally it is 2.5 liters per minute. Even if the rate of setting is

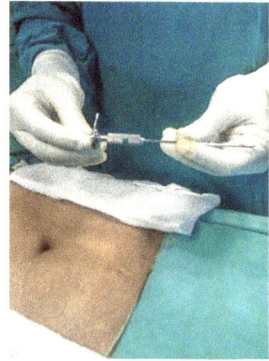

Fig. 5.1: Spring action of the Veress needle being checked

kept on the higher side, it is limited by the diameter and the lateral hole in the stylet (Figs 5.3 and 5.4).

The patency of the Veress needle is checked with the help of a 10 mL syringe filled with saline. The spring action of the Veress needle is checked by pressing the blunt tip against any hard surface. The umbilicus is the most commonly chosen point of insertion of the Veress needle as this is the thinnest part of the anterior abdominal wall. All the fasciae come and coalesce here.

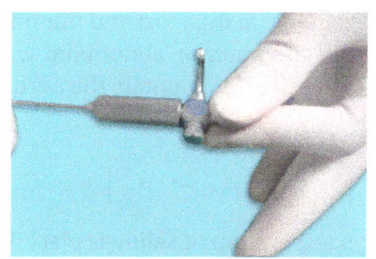

Fig. 5.2: Closed valve of Veress needle

A curvilinear incision of 2 mm is made at the lower margin of the umbilicus till the fascia is reached. The Veress needle is held in the dominant hand of the surgeon at an angle of 45° to the anterior abdominal wall with the ulnar aspect of the hand guarding against the inadvertent entry of the needle. The lower part of the anterior abdominal wall is lifted with the aid of the assistant. Two levels of resistance are encountered in the process, one at the level of fascia and the second at the level of the peritoneum. A 'give way' sensation is appreciated on entry into the peritoneum accompanied by a 'click' sound. Insufflations should be initiated on entry into the peritoneal cavity. Initially, the rate of flow will be 4-5 liters and once the set pressure of 14 mm Hg is reached, the flow is stopped. The rate of flow of CO_2 is decided by the diameter of the Veress needle, which is normally, 2.5 L/min. Normally, 2.5-3 L of CO_2 is sufficient for filling the peritoneal cavity. There is uniform distention of the abdomen.

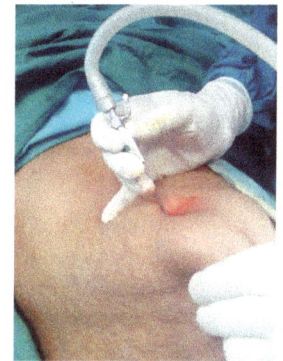

Fig. 5.3: Veress needle being introduced into the peritoneal cavity. The lower part of the abdominal wall being lifted. The ulnar aspect of right-hand guards the inadvertent entry of the Veress needle

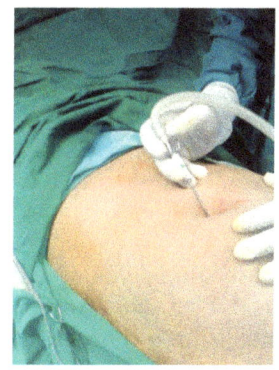

Fig. 5.4: Gas being insufflated. Uniform distension of abdominal wall

The obliteration of liver dullness confirms the intraperitoneal position of the needle.

The Veress needle is now taken out and the incision is enlarged to 10 mm. A sharp, pyramidal tip trocar is inserted with 45° angulation to the anterior abdominal wall with the tip directed toward the pelvic brim with twisting movements at the wrist and minimal pressure. During this process, the lower part of the anterior abdominal wall is kept lifted. A 'give way' sensation is felt after the trocar enters the peritoneal cavity. CO_2 is then connected to the trocar.

Confirmation of the Position

Drop test: A drop of saline is placed on top of the Veress needle and the abdominal cavity is slightly elevated, saline is sucked into the peritoneal cavity due to negative intraperitoneal pressure (Fig. 5.5).[3,4]

Percussion: There is uniform distension of the abdomen and if the needle is in position then percussion of the abdomen is resonant (Figs 5.6 and 5.7).

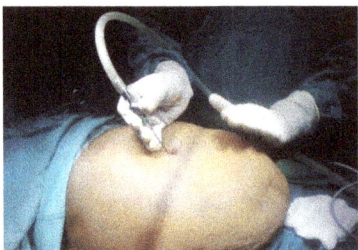

Fig. 5.5: Uniform distension of the abdominal wall

Aspiration: A partially filled syringe is used to aspirate, if there is egress of bowel contents, blood or urine then the needle is in bowel, vessel or bladder.

Instillation: About 5 mL of saline in the peritoneal cavity if the needle is in proper position then the saline flows freely. If the tip is in the abdominal wall then the fluid can be aspirated back.

Movement: If the needle is in position then it can be moved freely for a short distance in and out.

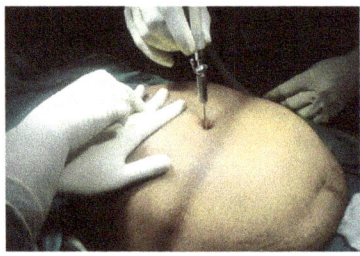

Fig. 5.6: Resonant to percussion

Direct Trocar Insertion

Direct trocar insertion technique was developed in order to reduce the various complications associated with Veress needle use such as failed insertion, preperitoneal insertion, intestinal injury and CO_2 embolism.[5] It is faster than the other methods of laparoscopic entry (Figs 5.8 to 5.10).[6]

It is a blind technique where a 5–10 mm subumbilical incision is made. The lower abdomen is lifted with the aid of an assistant and a trocar with a sharp pyramidal tip is introduced blindly.[7] The tip of the trocar should be directed to

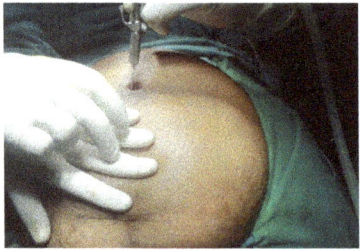

Fig. 5.7: Resonant to percussion

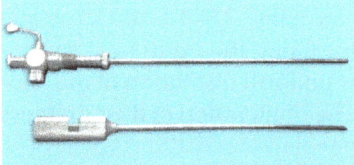

Fig. 5.8: Stylet and cannula of Veress needle

Peritoneal Access

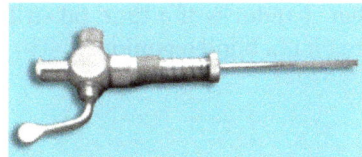

Fig. 5.9: Stylet with spring

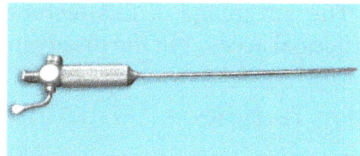

Fig. 5.10: Veress needle

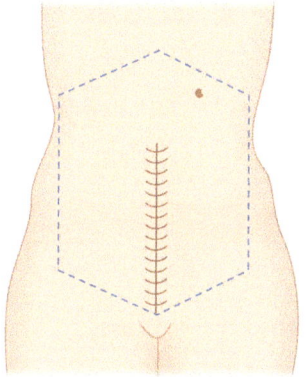

Fig. 5.11: Lower midline scar: Trocar is inserted in the Palmer's point

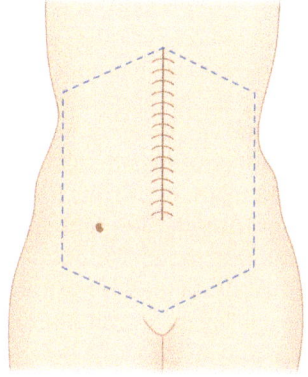

Fig. 5.12: Upper midline scar: Trocar is inserted in the right iliac fossa

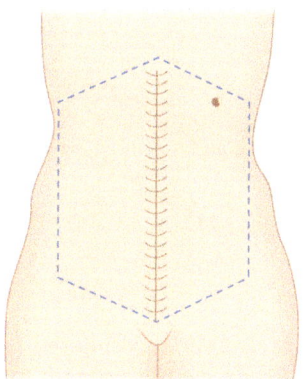

Fig. 5.13: Midline scar: Trocar is inserted in the Palmer's point

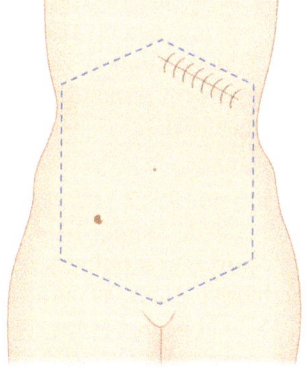

Fig. 5.14: Left subcoastal scar: Trocar is inserted either in the umbilicus or in right iliac fossa

the pelvic rim with twisting movements at the wrist. The pressure of insertion should be controlled with maximum thrust on the twisting movement.[8] A 'give way' sensation indicates entry into the peritoneal cavity. At no point should the direction of entry be kept downwards (vertical) as this increases the chance of injury to the bowel and major vascular structures (Figs 5.11 to 5.14).

The advantage of this technique is that it reduces the time taken for peritoneal access but the disadvantage is that it is a blind technique.[9]

Open Technique

Both the Veress needle and the first trocar entry are blind, therefore the chances of injury to the internal organs increases. To prevent such inadvertent injury, open access was introduced by Hasson.[10] Hasson cannula (Figs 5.15 to 5.17) has three components; a cone shaped sleeve, a metal cannula and a blunt-tipped obturator. On the conical sleeve there are two struts for affixing two fascial sutures.[11] The conical sleeve will slide on the metal cannula. Cannula is held in place by passing sutures through the fascial layers of the abdominal wall. This creates an effective seal, so that the pneumoperitoneum is maintained.

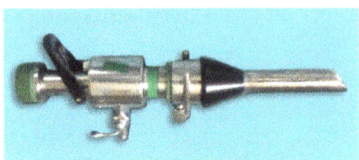

Fig. 5.15: Hasson cannula

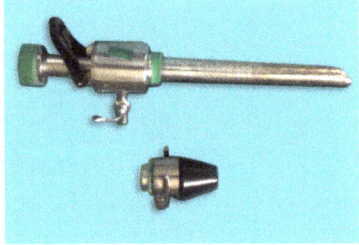

Fig. 5.16: Hasson cannula with the sleeve dismantled

Small 2 cm incision is made just below the umbilicus skin and the subcutaneous tissue is retracted to visualize the fascia. The fascia is incised horizontally and two stay sutures are taken. The peritoneum and the extraperitoneal fat are incised. The Hasson trocar is inserted under vision and stay suture tied.

Palmer's technique: The access was advocated by Palmer in 1940. Left upper quadrant (left subcoastal region) is known as Palmer's point, this point is used in case the umbilical entry is contraindicated.

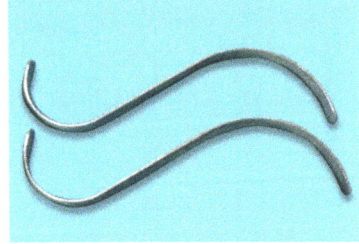

Fig. 5.17: 'S' retractors

This area is chosen because the adhesions are rarely encountered in this area. Splenomegaly should be ruled out. If necessary umbilical port may be introduced under vision.

■ REFERENCES

1. Harell AG, et al. Minimally invasive abdominal surgery: Lux, et al. Veritas past, present and future. Am J Surg. 2005;190(2):239-43.
2. Bruce V, MacFadyen Jr. Laparoscopic surgery of the abdomen, Laparoscopic Instrumentation. New York: Springer-Verleg; 2004. pp. 335-51.

3. Mishra RK. Textbook of Practical Laparoscopic Surgery, 3rd edition. Laparoscopic Equipment and Instrumentation. Jaypee Brothers Medical Publishers (P) Ltd; 2013. pp. 32-44.
4. Semm K. Tissue puncher and loop Ligation: new aids for surgical therapeutic laparoscopy. Endoscopic intra-abdominal surgery. Endoscopy. 1978;10(2):119-24.
5. Viols GA, Ternamian, et al. The Society of Obstetricians and Gynaecologists of Canada. Laparoscopic entry; a review of techniques, technologies and complications. J Obst Gyneco Can. 2007;29(5):433-65.
6. Byron JW, Markenson G, Miyazawa K. A randomized comparison of Veress needle and direct trocar insertion for laparoscopy. Surg Gynaecol Obstet. 1993;177(3):259-62.
7. Dingelder JR. Direct laparoscopic trocar insertion without prior pneumoperitoneum. J Reprod Med. 1978;21:45-7.
8. Theodoropou K, et al. Direct trocar insertion technique alternative for creation of pneumoperitoneum. JSLS. 2008;12:156-8.
9. Agresta F. Direct trocar insertion for laparoscopy. JSLS. 2012;16(2):252-9.
10. Hasson HM. Open laparoscopy versus closed laparoscopy: A comparison of complication rates. Adv Plan Parenthood. 1978;13(3):41-50.
11. Hasson HM. A modified instrument and method for laparoscopy. Am J Obst Gyneco. 1971;110(6):886-7.

CHAPTER 6

Electrocautery

NEWER ENERGY SOURCES

Electrocautery

In direct current, during electrocautery, current does not enter the patient's body, only the heated wire comes in contact with tissue and uses direct current. Electric current heats an instrument: clinical effect is realized when the heated tool is applied to tissue.

Electrosurgery

Alternating current, high frequency electric current passed through tissue to create a desired clinical effect; uses alternating current. In electrosurgery, the patient is included in the circuit and the current enters patient's body.

Circuit[1]

Circuit are the pathways for uninterrupted flow of electrons. Normally, electrons orbit the nuclei of atoms. Current flow occurs when electrons flow from one atom to the orbit of an adjacent atom.

Current: Rate of flow of electrons (Fig. 6.1) in a given period of time, measured in amperes (A).

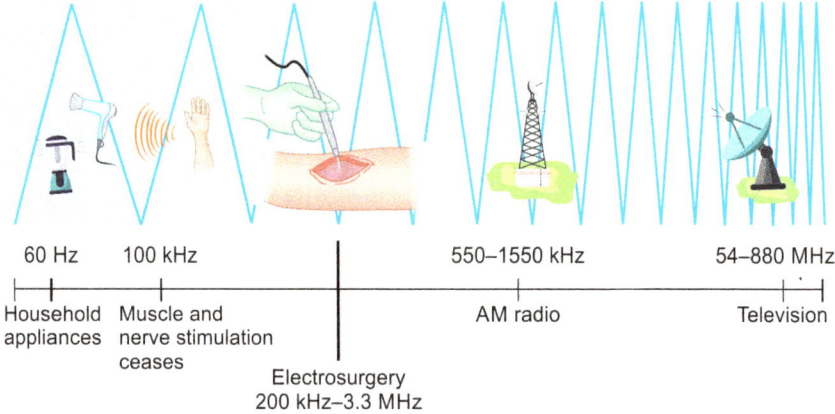

Fig. 6.1: Frequency of current (Am, amplitude modulation)

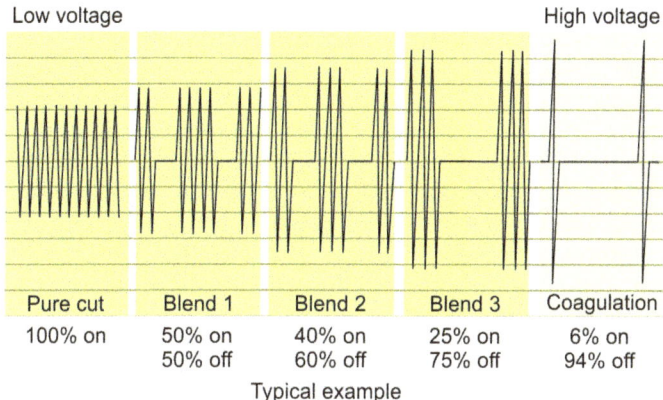

- High heat rapidly = Vaporization
- Low heat slowly = Coagulation
- Any waveform can do same function by modifying the other variable

Fig. 6.2: Voltage of current

Voltage: Electromagnetic force necessary to drive the current against resistance, measured in volts (V) (Fig. 6.2).

Resistance (impedance): Obstacle to the flow of current, measured in Ohms.

Ohm's law: Volt = Current X Resistance.

Standard electrical current has a frequency of 60 cycles per second (Hz). Electrosurgical systems could function at this frequency also, but the hazards are excessive neuromuscular stimulation and electrocution. Nerve and muscle stimulation cease when the frequency of the current reaches 100,000 cycles per second (100 kHz). Generator increases the frequency of current to 200,000 lakh per second (200 kHz/s), which can be used safely.

50°–80°C: Protein denaturation occurs.

Denaturation

The trihelical structure of the collagen is disrupted resulting in shrinkage of tissue. The cell walls rupture when the 100°–125°C Eschar formation occurs.

Monopolar Energy

In monopolar energy, the current flows from the generator to the patient through the active electrode. It reaches the generator (Fig. 6.3) through the return electrode. As the area of the active electrode is small than

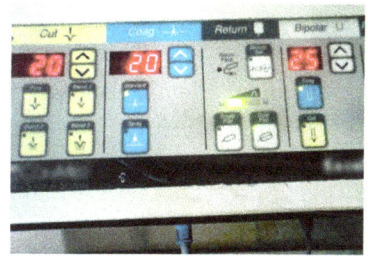

Fig. 6.3: Front panel of diathermy generator

the return electrode, current gets concentrated to produce the desired effect. The return electrode should have a surface of 143 cm^2 and should be coated with conductive gel.

The current output of the generators can be modulated to deliver two types of waveforms the so-called mode. The continuous mode of the current output is referred as 'cut' mode. The interrupted mode of current delivery is referred as 'coagulation' mode. In this mode, the time the tissue is exposed to the current is significantly reduced to approximately 6% of the time relative to the continuous cut mode.

Fulguration

At the time of fulguration lateral spread of energy is more than depth. It produces superficial eschar with minimal depth of necrosis. Practically, this happens when the coagulation paddle is pressed and the active electrode is held at a distance from the tissue.

Desiccation

Desiccation takes place when the active electrode is in contact with the tissue. No sparks are created and the heat generated in the tissue result in drying of the cells. This is the common electrosurgical effect used by the surgeons.

Blend

Blend provides both coagulation and cutting at the same time. Pure cutting mode provides excellent cutting, but poor hemostasis. Pure coagulation provides excellent homeostasis, but minimal cutting. Blend is alteration in the duty cycle from 100% cutting to 50% (blend 1) 40% (blend 2) and 25% (blend 3). The coagulation current is not altered, but decreasing cutting current provides cooling effect.

Cutting Current

Cutting current is continuous wave, high frequency and low voltage current. It produces rapid tissue heating with minimal associated coagulation, therefore no hemostasis. Cutting is a non-contact activity in which the active electrode is short distance from the tissue.

Coagulation current: Pulsed waveform, low frequency, high voltage current. In this, current is on 6% of the time and off for 94% of the time.

Monopolar Electrosurgery

- The circuit consists of the generator, active electrode, patient and patient return electrode
- The patient's tissue provides the impedance, producing heat

- Active electrode is in the wound
- Return electrode is elsewhere on the patient
- Current must flow through the patient.

In bipolar electrosurgery, one of the prongs acts as active electrode and the other acts as a return electrode. They are separated by few millimeters. The current passes only in tissue between the two prongs. It does not pass through the patient's body as in monopolar surgery (Figs 6.4 to 6.6).

Before 1970s, the generators were not isolated. In this situation, if the patient comes in contact with either say electrocardiogram (ECG) pad or IV stand, the current would flow through them, i.e. the path of least resistance.

Alternate Site Burns

The ECG electrode provided the path of least resistance to ground. However, it does not disperse the current over a large enough area. The heat produced an alternate site burn under the ECG electrode due to current concentration (Fig. 6.7).

Isolated Electrosurgical System

- Technology developed in 1968; eliminates hazard of current division/split
- Circuit is completed by generator, not ground
- Current does not recognize grounded objects as pathways

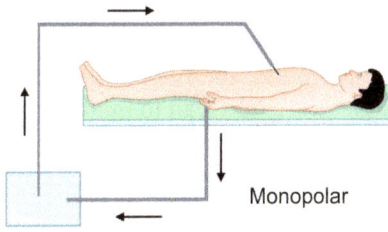

Fig. 6.4: Circuit of monopolar diathermy

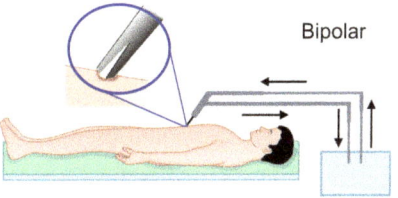

Fig. 6.5: Bipolar—active and return electrodes are in the prong

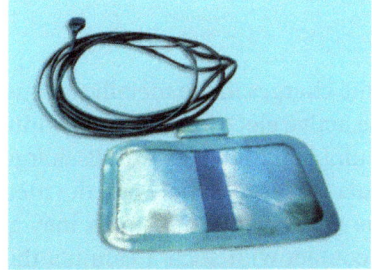

Fig. 6.6: Patient plate

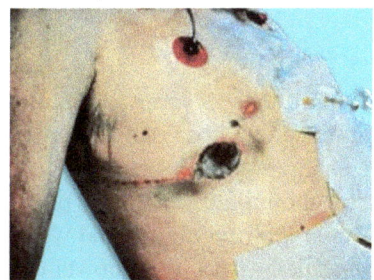

Fig. 6.7: Burns at the electrocardiogram (ECG) lead site

- Return electrode is the preferred pathway (Fig. 6.8).

Before 1970, the generators were not isolated from the ground. The advantage of isolation is current flows from the electrode to the patient return plate, which offers the path of least resistance from the patient to the generator.[2]

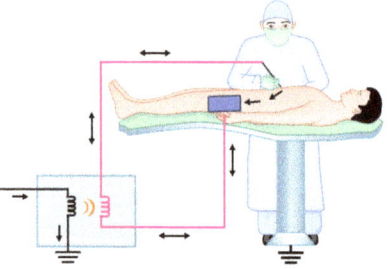

Fig. 6.8: Isolated electrosurgical system

Insulation Failure[3]

Normally, the laparoscopic hand instruments are insulated except at the tip, if the continuity of the sheath is lost due to overuse or due to repeated cleaning and sterilization, insulation failure occurs.[4] As shown in Figure 6.9, during laparoscopic surgery only the tip of the instrument is seen while the shaft for the most part is not under visualization. This may lead to injury to intra-abdominal organs such as bowel, which may go unnoticed during the time of surgery.

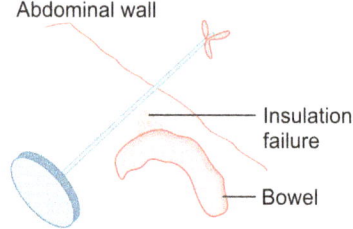

Fig. 6.9: Insulation failure

Direct Coupling

Direct coupling may occur that the active electrode in one hand may inadvertently touch a metal object in the other hand, such as the telescope, which in turn may be in contact with bowel. This could lead to injury to the bowel through the phenomenon called direct coupling.

Technical Pearl

Do not activate the generator when the active electrode is near another metal instrument or in the air (no tissue contact).

Capacitive Coupling

Normally, there is some accumulation of the charges in the metallic cannula that is used in laparoscopic surgery, as the active electrode and the cannula are separated by the insulation. The accumulated charges are discharged in the abdominal wall, but a plastic cannula is placed in between the metal cannula and the abdominal wall then the charges in the cannula may get accumulated and if the bowel comes in contact with such a cannula then there is injury to the bowel (Fig. 6.10). Here, the metal cannula and the abdominal wall are separated by a plastic sleeve (Figs 6.11 and 6.12).

Electrocautery

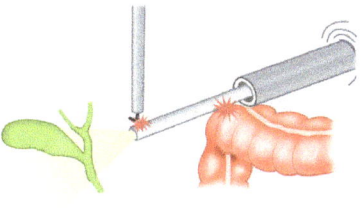

Fig. 6.10: Bowel injury

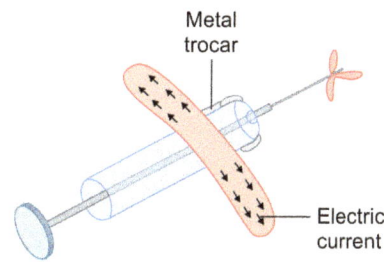

Fig. 6.11: Normal movement of charges

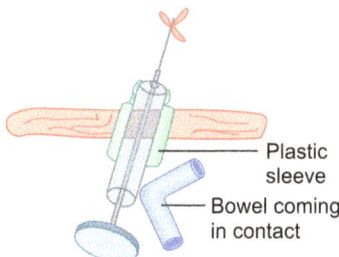

Fig. 6.12: Capacitive coupling—bowel injury

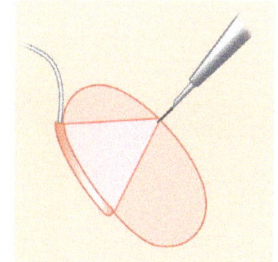

Fig. 6.13: Correct placement of return electrode

Return Electrode

The function of the return electrode is to remove the current safely from the patient's body. Return electrode burns occur when the heat produced is not safely dissipated by the size or conductivity of the return electrode. Concentration of electrons at the active electrode creates heat, whereas, dispersion of current at the return electrode causes less heat (Figs 6.13 and 6.14).

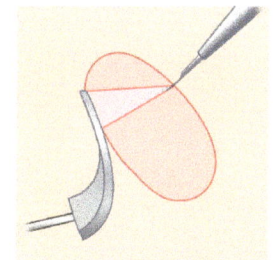

Fig. 6.14: Incorrect placement of return electrode

Ideal Return Pad

- Large surface area
- Close to the operative site
- Surface area impedance is increased by adhesive failure, excessive hair, bony prominences, adipose tissue, wet surfaces and scar tissue
- Peripheral adhesive layer for firm contact with the patient's body and prevent contact with moisture due to spillage or soiling of area.

REFERENCES

1. Massarweh NN, et al. Electrosurgery: History, principles and current and future uses. J Am Coll Surg. 2006;202(3):520-30.
2. Moak E. Electrosurgical unit safety. The role of perioperative nurse. AORNJ. 1991;53:744-52.
3. C Palanivelu. Art of Laparoscopic Surgery Textbook and Atlas. Laparoscopic Hemostasis, 1st edition, New Delhi: Jaypee Brothers Medical Publishers (P) Ltd; 2007. pp. 69-84.
4. Vacaville TG. Electrosurgery at laparoscopy: guidelines to avoid complications. Gynaec Endoscopy. 1994;3:143-50.

CHAPTER 7

Harmonic and Vessel Sealing Device

The handpiece incorporates the transducer and is connected to the generator through an electric cable. The ferroelectric ceramic crystals of the transducer vibrate (expand and contract) and produce ultrasound waves. The transducer is able to transform the electric signal into mechanical motion. The vibrations are conducted through a metal rod to the tip of the instrument (Figs 7.1 to 7.4).[1]

The harmonic scalpel (Figs 7.5 and 7.6) works at a lower temperature than the electrosurgical devices, since it denatures proteins by mechanically breaking down the hydrogen bonds in protein molecules when the blade vibrates at 55.5 kHz.[2] The temperature never exceeds 80°C, the tissue charring effect is nill.[3]

Harmonic scalpel leads to short duration of surgery, less lateral thermal damage and perhaps the greatest advantage that no current passes through the body.[4]

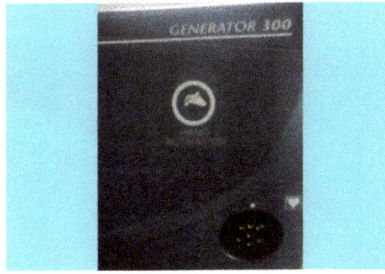

Fig. 7.1: Generator with cable socket

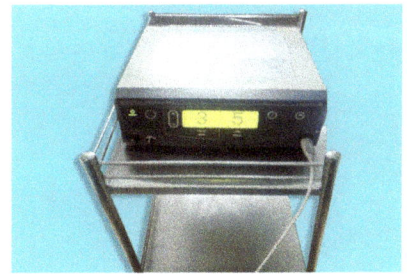

Fig. 7.2: Generator with cable plugged in

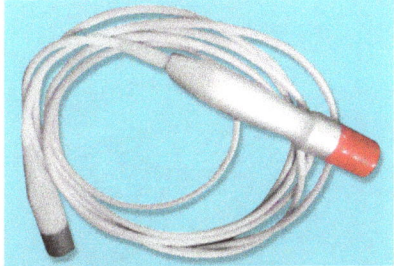

Fig. 7.3: Electric cable, which connects the generator to the handpiece

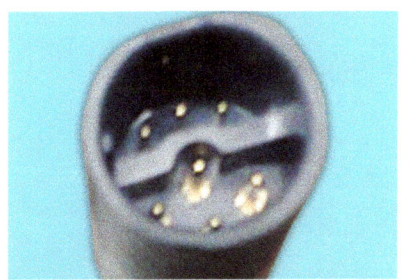

Fig. 7.4: Generator end of the electric cable

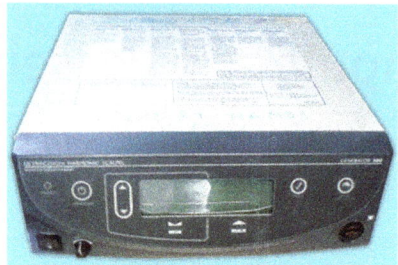

Fig. 7.5: Harmonic generator

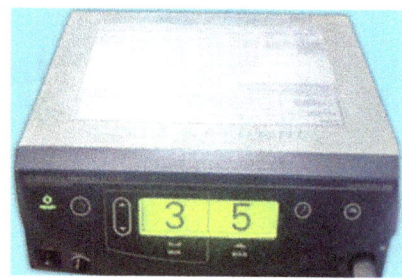

Fig. 7.6: Harmonic (minimum and maximum reading)

Another potential advantage is superior visualization, as there is no smoke compared with electrically activated devices.[5]

ULTRASONIC SHEARS (HARMONIC)

- Hemostasis by coaptive coagulation at lower temperature ranging from 50 to 100°C
- Electromagnetic energy from dedicated generator
- Handpiece (Figs 7.7 to 7.10)
- Piezoelectric transducer disks (acoustic assembly)
- Sine waves to the blade
- Mechanical vibration
- Drives active blade at 55.5 kHz/s

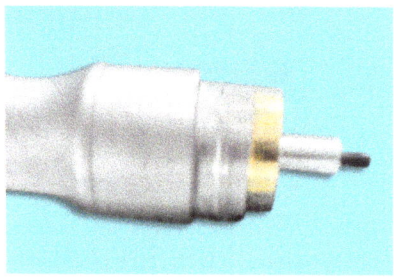

Fig. 7.7: Handpiece end of the cable

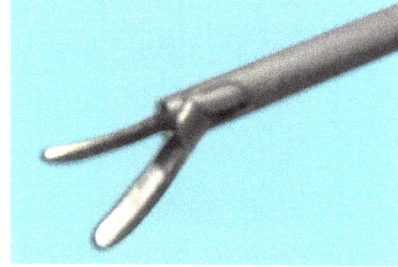

Fig. 7.8: Effector end of handpiece

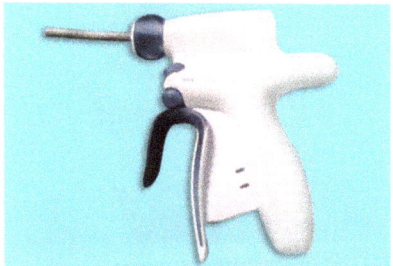

Fig. 7.9: Handpiece

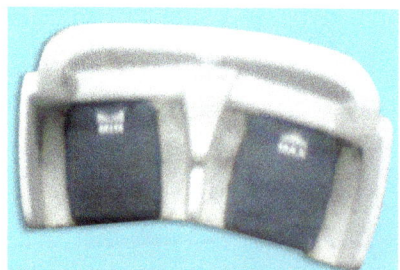

Fig. 7.10: Foot pedal

- Vibrating blade contact + pressure = coaptation (adherence) of blood vessel (collapse of collagen molecules)
- The tip of ultrasonic shears has two portions a stationary side that supports the grasped tissue and vibratory side that transmits the ultrasonic energy to the tissues.

Four Basic Effects

1. Coaptation and pressure
2. *Coagulation (after above):* Vaporization and protein denaturation
3. *Cutting:* Combination of tension and pressure rapidly stretches tissue till elastic limit; sawing mechanism of blade cuts
4. *Cavitation (occurs as side effect):* Vapor bubbles at body temperature in surrounding tissue—aids dissection of tissue planes; enhances visibility in operative field, especially near vital structures.

Benefits of Harmonic Devices

- Used for sealing vessels up to including 3–4 mm
- Minimal lateral thermal tissue damage
- Simultaneous cutting and coagulation of soft tissue and vessels
- Minimal charring and desiccation
- Fewer instrument exchanges to simplify procedure steps
- No electricity passes to or through the patient
- Safer dissection near vital structures
- Minimal smoke for improved visibility in the surgical field
- Compared to clamp, cut and tie
- Compared to electrocautery.

BIPOLAR VESSEL SEALING DEVICE

Bipolar vessel sealing device applies a precise amount of mechanical pressure and radiofrequency energy. There is fusion of the opposing layers of the vessel due to denaturing of the collagen and elastin,[6] which can be transected.[2] There is denaturation of the proteins thus truly sealing the vessels. Its lateral thermal spread is less than 1 mm.[7] It is a feedback controlled sealing system that seals vessels up to 7 mm in diameter. The posterior jaw is coated and insulated.

LigaSure is used in major surgeries such as splenectomy,[8] pancreaticoduodenectomy,[9] liver resections,[10] colectomy,[11] donor nephrectomy.[12]

REFERENCES

1. Boni L, Benevento A, Cantore F, et al. Technological advances in minimal invasive surgery. Expert Rev Med Devices. 2006;3(2):147-53.
2. Druzijanic, et al. Comparison of lateral thermal damage of the human peritoneum using monopolar diathermy, harmonic scalpel and LigaSure. Can J Surg. 2012;55(5):317-21.

3. Gill BS, MacFadney B V Jr. Ultrasonic dissectors and minimally invasive surgery. Semin Laparosc Surg. 1999;6(4):229-34.
4. Emam TA, Cuschieri A. How safe is high-power ultrasonic dissection? Ann Surg. 2003;237(2):186-91.
5. Payne JH. Ultrasonic dissection. Surg Endos. 1994;8(5):416-18.
6. Thompson S, Pearce JA, Kennedy JS. Mechanisms of electrosurgical fusion for large vessel hemostasis. Minim Invasive Ther Allied Technol. 1995;4:19.
7. Sartori PV, DeFinas, Colombo G, et al. LigaSure versus ultracision in thyroid surgery: a prospective randomized study. Langenbecks Arch Surg. 2008;393(5):655-8.
8. Romano F, Caprotti R, Franciosi C, et al. Laparoscopic splenectomy using LigaSure. Preliminary experience. Surg Endosc. 2002;16(11):1608-11.
9. Belli G, Fantini C, Ciciliano F. Pancreaticoduodenectomy in portal hypertension: use of the LigaSure. J Hepatobiliary Pancreat Surg. 2003;10(3):215-7.
10. Romanio F, et al. Hepatic surgery using the LigaSure vessel sealing system. World J Surg. 2005;29(1):110-2.
11. Araki Y, Noake T, Kanazawa M, et al. Clipless hand-assisted. Laparoscopic total colectomy using LigaSure Atlas. Kurume Med J. 2004;51(2):105-8.
12. Constant DL, Florman SS, Medez F, et al. Use of the LigaSure vessel sealing device in laparoscopic living-donor nephrectomy. Transplantation. 2004;78(11):1661-4.

CHAPTER 8

Homeostasis and Suturing

HOMEOSTASIS AND SUTURING TECHNIQUE

Suture Material

The conventional suture materials and needles are used in laparoscopy. Approximately, 10 cm of suture is required for the initial suture and additional 2 cm for each suture. This should be instructed to the scrub nurse or else long length of suture material intracorporeally is very cumbersome and frustrating. The suture material, which is easily handled is Vicryl.

Needle holder should have a coaxial handle and a locking mechanism. Coaxial handles are better than the pistol handle as there is less strain on the hand and greater maneuverability. They should be strong with heavy handle. The tip is usually tapered with single moving jaw. Tip may be either straight or curved.

Ski needles have been used in laparoscopic surgery as they have a curved tip with straight shaft. All conventional needles that are used in open surgery can be used in laparoscopic surgery. To take them inside the abdominal cavity they may be temporarily straightened. Swaged needles are to be used (Fig. 8.1).

Ergonomics

The camera port is in the center, and the right- and left- hand ports are on either side. This will give a triangulation effect at the tip of the instruments, which is vital.[1] The instruments should meet at an angle of 60°–70° for effective suturing. If the angle is less than this then there will be overcrowding and sword fighting of the instruments. If the angle is wider, then there will be straining of the hands.

The endoscope to target tissue distance is 7.5–15 cm longer time was taken and the performance quality deteriorated, when the distance was decreased to 5 cm.[2]

Passage of Needle into the Abdominal Cavity

The 10 mm reducing sleeve is used to take the needle inside the abdominal cavity. The thread is loaded in a reverse direction into the sleeve by holding the thread 1 cm away from the needle. The reducer is introduced in the

48 Homeostasis and Suturing

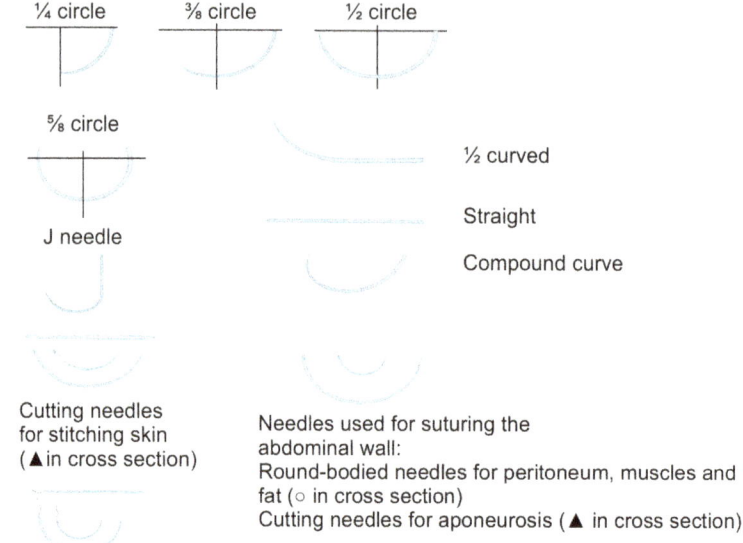

Fig. 8.1: Types of needles used for sutures. The sutures are swaged on to prevent a shoulder and allow easy passage through tissues

peritoneal cavity. It is better to take smaller needle for the purpose, if larger needles have to be taken than they have to be straightened.

Another way of introducing the needle into the abdominal cavity is by directly puncturing the abdominal wall. The needle is then pulled into the abdominal cavity under vision. This is done in thin individuals.

In third method, one of the trocar is removed and a 5 mm instrument carries the thread along with the needle into the abdominal cavity. Similar method can be employed for removal of the needle.

Loading of the Needle

Needle is placed over the tissue with the sharp tip facing towards the left. The static jaw of the needle holder is placed below the needle and the moving jaw is gently closed with slight downward pressure over the tissues. The needle gets positioned itself at right angles, then the needle is held firmly. The optimum angle is more than 90° and the point of holding is at the junction of middle and proximal third.[3]

Adjusting the Needle

The needle holder has to be rotated in all directions in order to make sure the needle is perpendicular to the needle holder. If the tip faces the surgeon then the grip on the needle is released and with the left hand the needle is gently manipulated to make it right angled[4] by adjusting the needle to right angle, with the left hand (Fig. 8.2).

Intracorporeal Knotting and Suturing: Square Knot

After taking the bite, the thread is held at 6 cm distal to the exit point. The thread is taken towards the tail to form a loop. Then the right-hand instrument is used to under wrap the thread and the tail is pulled to form a half knot (Figs 8.3 and 8.4). Again the loop is formed and an over wrap is done, and the tail is pulled to complete the square knot (Figs 8.5 to 8.7).

Endoloop

Application of the Endoloop

Endoloops (Fig. 8.8) are used to ligate the pedicles. They are commercially available loops, but the indigenously made loops are cheaper, they have a slip knot and Roeder's knot is widely used one (Fig. 8.9). The loop is passed into the abdominal cavity usually through the right-hand working port and is placed around the structure (tissue) to be looped. The left-hand grasper holds the tissue and pulls out of the loop. This is then held by the assistant to give slight tension, while applying the knot by the surgeon. The thread is held by the right hand and the plastic knot pusher is pushed towards the pedicle to tighten the loop. The plastic knot pusher is removed and the thread is cut by the scissors.

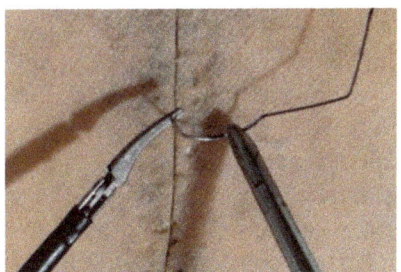

Fig. 8.2: Adjusting the needle to right angle, with the left hand

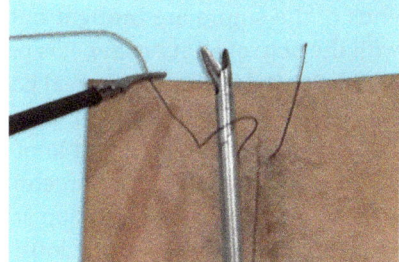

Fig. 8.3: Under wrap

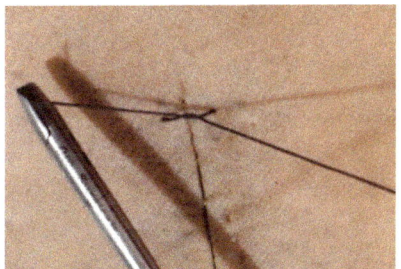

Fig. 8.4: First half knot formed

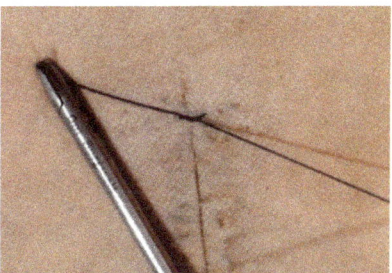

Fig. 8.5: Tail being pulled

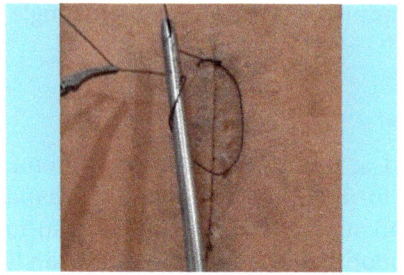

Fig. 8.6: Over wrap

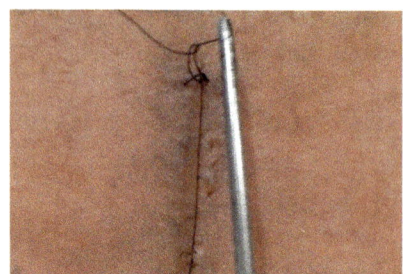

Fig. 8.7: Square knot completed

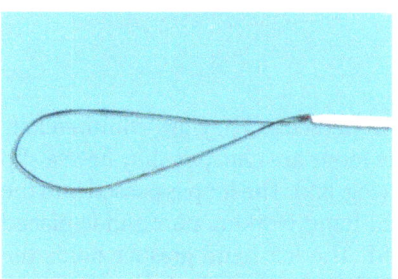

Fig. 8.8: Endoloop

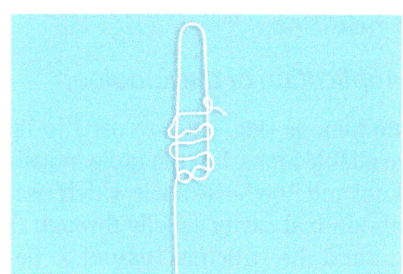

Fig. 8.9: Roeder's knot

Extracorporeal Knots

The suture material is passed around the structure to be ligated and both the ends of the suture are brought out through the trocar. Knot is created and with the help of knot pusher, it is passed intracorporeally. Roeder's knot this is widely used for extracorporeal knotting.

Loop is formed by passing the thread around the index finger of the assistant and then initial half knot is made. The knot is held by the thumb and the index finger of the surgeon. Three and half loops are passed in front over the two limbs. The last loop is passed on only one limb of the loop. The knot is tightened over the previously placed loops.

Staplers

Maximum gap: Measurement of the gap between the staple leg furthest from the backspan to the backspan (Figs 8.10A and B).

Minimum gap: Measurement of the gap between the staple leg closest to the backspan to the backspan.

Delta gap: The difference in measurement between maximum gap and minimum gap.

Twist: The height of farthest leg out of the plane of staple backspan (Fig. 8.11).

Advantage

The advantage with the staplers is that they reduce the time duration of the surgery.[5] They can be used when multiple anastomosis are required.

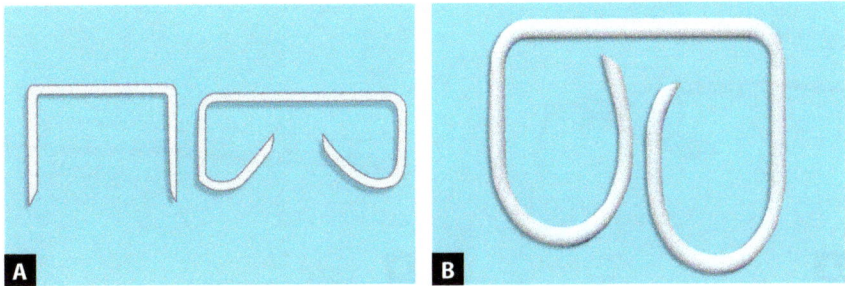

Figs 8.10A and B: (A) Staple configuration: Before firing; after firing; (B) Gap between staple leg and backspan.

Staplers place double-staggered row of titanium staples, which provides effective tissue closure. Staplers join tissues in a B-shaped configuration with a fine metal wire. As the stapler is fired, the open legs of the stapler are driven through the tissue and the staple resembles the shape of alphabet 'B'. The B shape will allow the small vessels to pass in between the legs thus allowing the viability of the tissue in between the staple line and the cut edge. Transient seepage of blood along the cut margin indicates adequate blood supply to tissue margin.[4] When the device is employed from within the lumen an inversion anastomosis is seen. The 12 mm ports are required for the introduction of endostaplers. When longer transaction is required multiple firings have to be done. Multifire endo GIA 30–45 places six staggered rows, and divides the tissue between the third and fourth row.

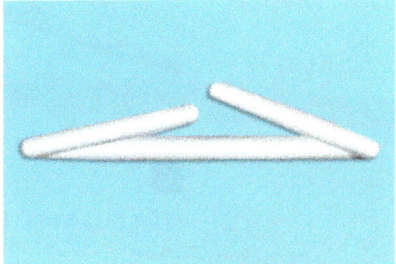

Fig. 8.11: Twist

Flexible or articulating linear staplers have an articulating component in between the body and jaw (Figs 8.12A to C to 8.18A to C). This helps particularly in pelvis, such as in anterior resection.

Circular staplers
Circular staplers place the staples in a circular fashion in double-staggered rows. They are available in various sizes. The various diameters available are 21, 25, 29 and 33 mm. The internal diameters are 12.5, 16.5, 20.5, 24.5 mm respectively. The shaft may be straight or curved. The 21 and 25 mm diameters are chosen for esophagus, and 29 and 33 mm diameter are chosen for rectum.

They have a detachable anvil, which is placed in the proximal bowel with the help of purse string suture (Figs 8.19 to 8.22A to C).

The stapling device is introduced through the anus. The spike in the head of the device is advanced, while a grasper is used to push the distal bowel, to prevent the tear in the bowel. The spike is advanced through the staple line in the distal bowel till it is completely out.

52 Homeostasis and Suturing

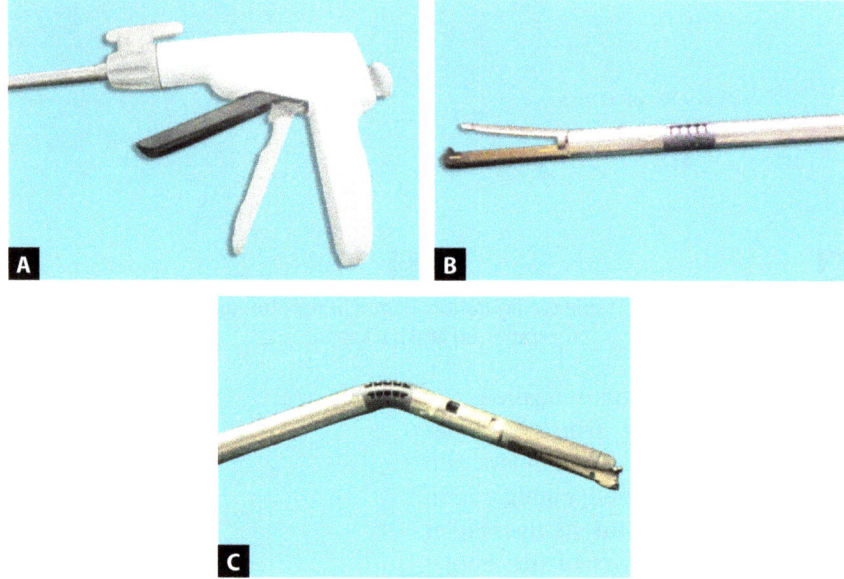

Figs 8.12A to C: Endoscopic linear cutter

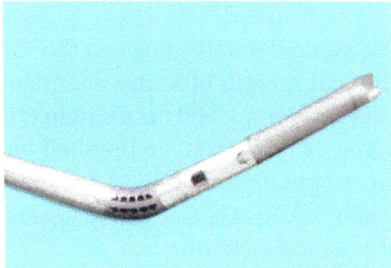

Fig. 8.13: Endoscopic linear cutter flex roticulator

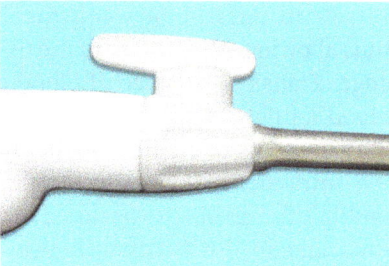

Fig. 8.14: Endoscopic linear cutter flex roticulator knob

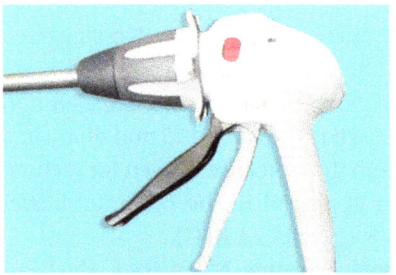

Fig. 8.15: Echelon flex 60 roticulator

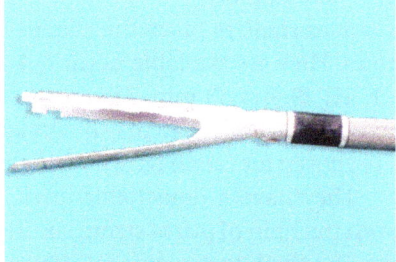

Fig. 8.16: Echelon 60

The anvil is engaged to the stapling device and twisting of the bowel is looked for. The anvil is approximated to the device and tightened, then the device is fired. Finally, the handle is turned anticlockwise to dislodge the stapler and removed gently. The anvil is looked for two intact doughnuts (Figs 8.23 to 8.25).

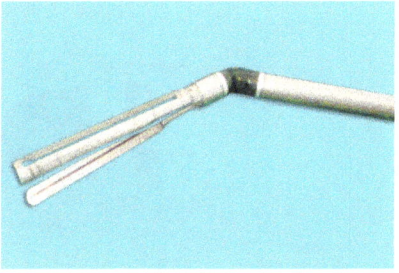

Fig. 8.17: Echelon roticulator

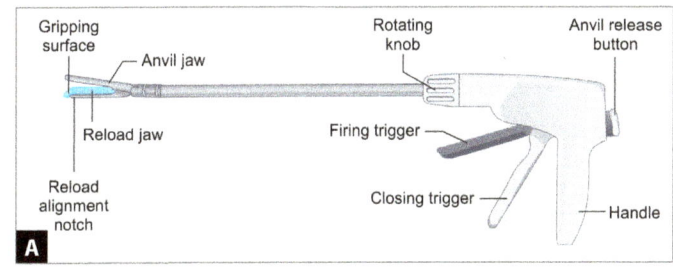

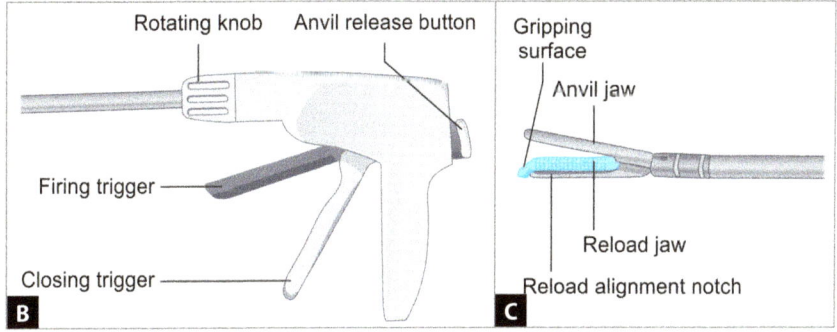

Figs 8.18A to C: Endoscopic linear cutter

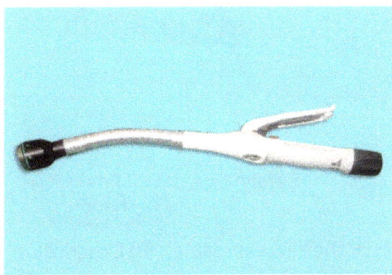

Fig. 8.19: Curved circular stapler

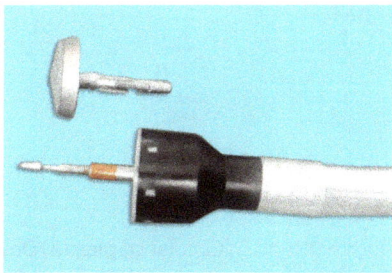

Fig. 8.20: Anvil separated from the shaft

54 Homeostasis and Suturing

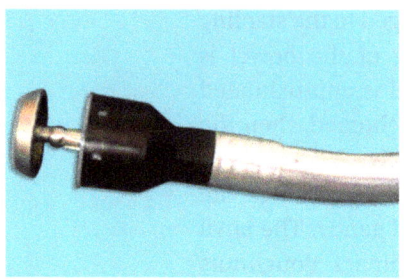

Fig. 8.21: Anvil in position

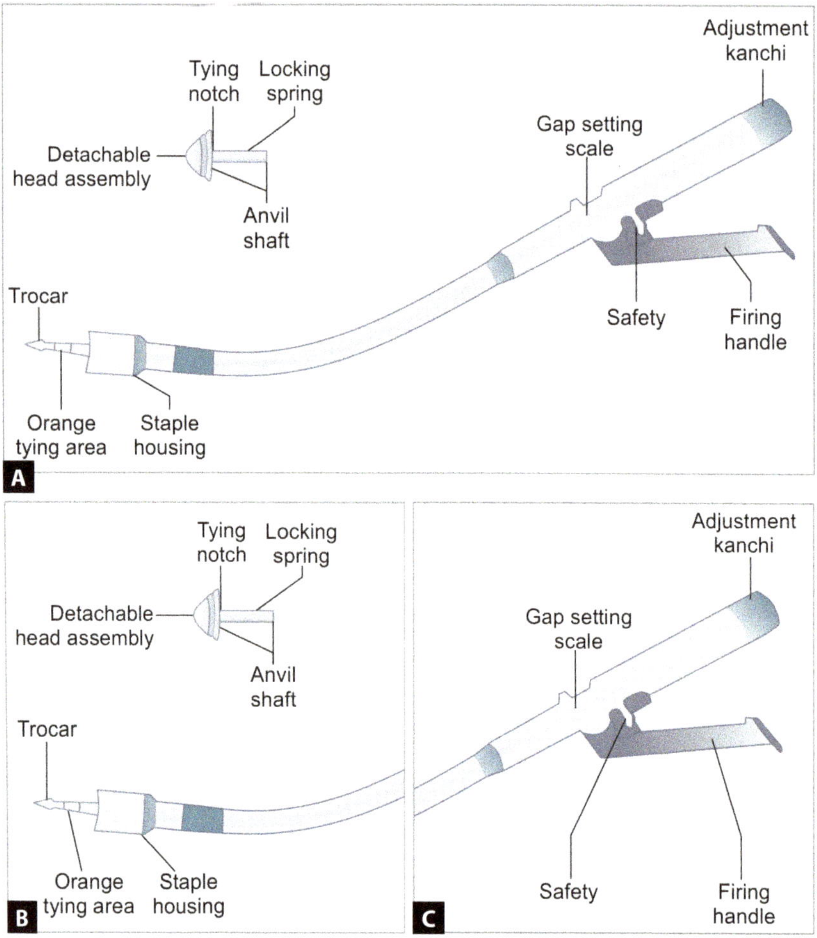

Figs 8.22A to C: Circular stapler. (A) Description of the circular stapler; (B) Description of anvil end; (C) Handle description.

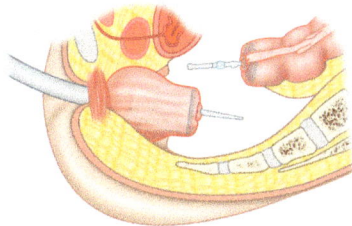

Fig. 8.23: Purse string around the anvil with shaft through the anus

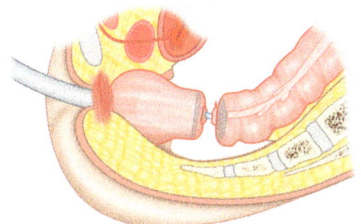

Fig. 8.24: Joining of the anvil and the retainer

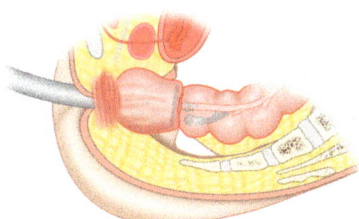

Fig. 8.25: Removal of the stapler

REFERENCES

1. Joice P, Hanna GB, Cuschieri A. Ergonomic evaluation of laparoscopic bowel suturing. Am J Surg. 1998;176(4):373-8.
2. Hanna GB, Shimi S, Cuschieri A. Influence of direction of view, target-to-endoscope distance and manipulation angle on endoscopic knot tying. Br J Surg. 1997;84(10):1460-4.
3. Szabo Z, Hunter J, Berci G, et al. Analysis of surgical movements during suturing in laparoscopy. Endosc Surg Allied Technol. 1994;2(1):55-61.
4. C Palanivelu. Art of Laparoscopic Surgery: Textbook and Atlas, 1st edition. Laparoscopic Tissue Approximation. New Delhi: Jaypee Brothers Medical Publishers (P) Ltd; 2007. pp. 85-109.
5. Bruce v Mac Fadeye. Laparoscopic surgery of the abdomen. Laparoscopic Instrumentation. New York: Springer-Verleg; 2004. pp. 335-51.

CHAPTER 9

Troubleshooting and Complications

TROUBLESHOOTING IN LAPAROSCOPY AND REMEDIES (Table 9.1)

Table 9.1: Troubleshooting in laparoscopy

Problems	Causes	Remedies
Loss of pneumoperitoneum	Stopcock open	Close the stopcock
	Leak from the cap	Change the cap (wiser)
	Excessive suction	Suck when the tip is in fluid
	Loose connection of the insufflator tube	Tighten the connection
	Loss of gas from the sides of trocar	Secure with sutures
Excessive pressure required for insufflation	Veress needle not in the peritoneal cavity	Reinsert the Veress needle
	Kinking of the tube	Straighten the tube
	Inadequate muscle relaxation	Muscle relaxation to be increased
Inadequate lighting	Lose connection either at the source or at the scope	Fix it properly
	Bulb is burnt	Replace bulb
	Fiber optics damaged	Light cable to be replaced
	Reduce monitor brightness	Adjust setting
Poor quality picture	Fogging of lens	Clean the lens with warm saline, gently touching the solid organs
	Condensation on the eyepiece, camera lens	Cleaning the eyepiece of scope and camera before fixing
Flickering	Camera cable connecting plug moisture	Use compressed air to dry

Contd...

Contd...

Problems	Causes	Remedies
Blurred image	Incorrect focusing, cracked lens of scope and camera	Correct the focusing, replace the lens as required
	Blood in the peritoneal cavity	As blood absorbs light, it has to be suctioned
Poor suction	Blood clot in the suction cannula/tube	Clean the cannula/tube
Poor irrigation	Lid of the container is loose with connection of the irrigation tube	Tighten the container lid, connect the tube properly
Diathermy	Diathermy not working	Cable connection to be checked on both sides, foot paddle connection need to be checked
No picture on the monitor	Camera control unit not on	Make sure all the sockets are plugged, light source connected, cable should run from 'video out' on camera control unit (CCU) to 'video in' on monitor
Monitor too bright	Manual maximum, monitor brightness high	Change to automatic, readjust setting

■ COMPLICATIONS OF LAPAROSCOPY

1. *Trocar-associated complications:* Trocar-related complications arise, because of initial blind insertion. Adherent organs and bowel may be injured especially, if there are scars. The Hasson technique eliminates the complications associated with initial blind entry of Veress needle and trocar. All subsequent trocars should be inserted under direct vision, to avoid injury to the inferior epigastric vessels and the subsequent trocars should be inserted lateral to these vessels. Trocar site bleeding can be controlled by compression (tamponade) with the trocar, coagulation, suturing externally, Foley balloon tamponade, intracorporeal suturing and laparotomy.
2. *Bowel injury:* Patients who have had previous abdominal surgeries (scar) are more susceptible to bowel injuries. They have to be recognized immediately and repaired either laparoscopically or by laparotomy. The trocar needs to be left in place to identify the injury.
3. *Vascular injury:* Most of the injuries can be repaired with direct suturing.
4. *Bladder injury:* This may occur by the Veress needle or insertion of low trocar. The risk increases with previous abdominal surgeries. Injury to the bladder is suspected if there is blood in the urobag.

Whenever surgeries in the lower abdomen are planned, the best way to reduce injury to bladder is catheterization.

5. *Infection of the port site:* Occurs when the infected specimens come in contact with the skin and subcutaneous tissue, while retrieving specimen (appendix and gallbladder). These can be avoided if the retrieval is done in a plastic bag and also the port has to be cleaned with betadine solution. The problem is more with umbilicus as it contains lot of dirt, which has to be cleaned with a piece of wet gauze.
6. *Incisional hernia:* Defects larger than 10 mm should be closed with sutures.
7. *Subcutaneous emphysema:* This occurs when the tip of the Veress needle is not in the peritoneal cavity. Gas will travel along the fascial planes to the head neck, chest, groin, scrotum.[1] The affected areas are swollen and can be palpated as crepitus. Carbon dioxide (CO_2) is quickly absorbed within 24-48 hours.
8. Pneumothorax.
9. Pneumomediastinum.[2]

Avoiding Complications

Laparoscopic surgery requires various positions for surgery. The patient should be safely secured to the table to prevent fall when in extreme positions.[3] The risk of thromboembolic complications is higher when the duration of surgery increases and also with the use of pneumoperitoneum, the venous return from the lower limbs is reduced.[4,5] Intermittent sequential compression stockings lower the risk of postoperative deep vein thrombosis.[3] Anything that prevents the progression of the surgery should be a criteria for conversion. Exposure and visualization of the ureters in pelvic surgeries will minimize the potential for injury. In case of diverticulitis ureteral catheterization helps.

Bowel should always be handled with the bowel holding forceps and should never be locked. Tumor recurrence at the port site can be taken care of by retrieving the specimen in a bag. Intraperitoneal insufflations of CO_2 increases the arterial content of CO_2 by transperitoneal absorption, therefore continuous capnometry is required.[6,7]

REFERENCES

1. Haglund, et al. Complications related to pneumoperitoneum. In: Bailey RW, Flowers JL (Eds). St Louis: Quality Medical Publishing; 1995. p. 51.
2. Puri GD, Singh H. Ventilatory effects of laparoscopy under general anaesthesia. Br J Anaesth. 1992;68(2):211-3.
3. Schwenk W, Böhm B, Junghans T, et al. Intermittent sequential compression of the lower limbs prevents venous stasis in laparoscopic and conventional colorectal surgery. Dis Colon Rectum. 1997;40(9):1056-62.

4. Sibbald WJ, Paterson NA, Holliday RL, et al. The Trendelenburg position: hemodynamic effects in hypotensive and normotensive patients. Crit Care Med. 1979;7(5):218-24.
5. Diamant M, Benumof JL, Saidman LJ. Hemodynamics of increased intra-abdominal pressure: Interaction with hypovolemia and halothane anesthesia. Anesthesiology. 1978;48(1):23-7.
6. Kaplan MB, et al. Laparoscopic surgery: A View From the Head of the Table. Semin Laparosc Surg. 1994;1(4):207-10.
7. Beck de. Laparoscopic surgery. Complications of colon and rectal surgery. Balitmore: Williams & Wilkins; 2002. pp. 156-62.

CHAPTER 10

Laparoscopic Appendectomy

APPENDICITIS

Positions

The various positions of the appendix are retrocecal 74%, paracecal 2%, preileal 1%, postileal 1%, pelvic 21% and subileal 0.5%.

Anatomy of Appendix

At birth, the appendix is short and broad at its base, gradually it attains its tubular structure. The position of the base of the appendix is constant, being found at the confluence of the three tenia coli.

Mesoappendix arises from the lower surface of the mesentery. Sometimes the terminal third of the appendix is bereft of mesoappendix. In childhood it is transparent and the vessels are easily seen. Appendicular artery is a branch of lower division of right ileocolic artery, and enters into the mesoappendix behind the terminal ileum. It lies in the free border of the mesoappendix (Fig. 10.1).

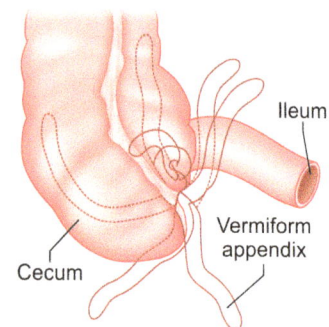

Fig. 10.1: Positions of the appendix

Etiology

One of the major etiological factors for the development of appendicitis is obstruction to the lumen of appendix. Fecolith is frequently implicated, which contains inspissated fecal material calcium phosphate, bacteria and epithelial debris. Bacterial proliferation involves both aerobic and anaerobic organisms.

Pathology

Lymphoid hyperplasia causes obstruction of the lumen. Once there is obstruction, continued mucus secretion and inflammatory exudates increase the intraluminal pressure leading to lymphatic obstruction. Resolution may occur at this stage. If the condition progresses then there is venous obstruction with bacterial invasion into the submucosa. This may progress to gangrene or perforation, peritonitis will occur if there is transmigration of the bacteria through the ischemic wall of the appendix.

Alternatively the omentum and the small intestine may become adherent to the inflamed appendix to form a mass. Omentum surrounds the inflamed appendix in order to prevent the spread of the infection to the surrounding organs that is why it is known as the 'policeman of the abdomen'.

McBurney's Point

McBurney's point is a point at the junction of medial two third and lateral one third of right spinoumbilical line. The base of the appendix corresponds to the McBurney's point. Maximum tenderness is in the McBurney's point in appendicitis. In the Figure 10.2, M is the McBurney's point and U is the umbilicus.

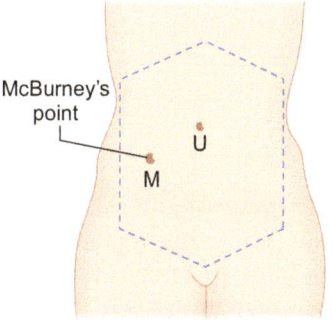

Fig. 10.2: McBurney's point (M) in relation to the umbilicus (U)

Symptoms[1]

- Periumbilical pain
- Shifting of pain to the right iliac fossa
- Anorexia
- Nausea and vomiting.

Shifting of pain: Initially, the pain is in the periumbilical region, which is associated with anorexia nausea and vomiting. This is midgut visceral discomfort as the appendix is a derivative of midgut. As the inflammation of the appendix progresses, the parietal peritoneum in the region gets irritated and the pain shifts to the right iliac fossa, the latter pain is more constant. Some patients notice the shift in the pain.

Signs

1. Pyrexia.
2. Tenderness in right iliac fossa.
3. Guarding and rigidity.
4. Rebound tenderness.
5. *Pointing sign:* The patient is asked to show the point of maximum pain and the shifting of pain. Palpation is started in the left iliac fossa and moved to the right iliac fossa in anticlockwise direction. Tenderness will be present at the McBurney's point.
6. *Rovsing's sign:* Deep palpation in the left iliac fossa causes pain in the right iliac fossa, due to movement of the intestine towards the right iliac fossa.

7. *Psoas sign:* When the inflamed appendix is in contact with the psoas muscle, this muscle will go into spasm and the patient flexes his/her right hip for relief of pain. Hyperextension of the hip joint will cause pain in the abdomen.
8. *Obturator sign:* Flexion and internal rotation of the hip causes pain if the inflamed appendix is in contact with the obturator internus due to spasm of this muscle.

Pelvic appendix will cause tenderness on rectal examination. Inflamed appendix when in contact with rectum may cause diarrhea and when in contact with the urinary bladder will cause frequency of micturition.

Differential Diagnosis

Children

- Gastroenteritis
- Meckel's diverticulitis
- Intussusception occurs due to weaning and hypertrophy of ileal lymphatics (medium age is 18 months)
- Mesenteric adenitis.

Males

1. Regional ileitis is indistinguishable, weight loss and diarrhea may be helpful. It may be nonspecific or due to Crohn's disease or *Yersinia pestis*.
2. *Right ureteric colic:* In this, the pain radiates from loin to groin, history of burning micturition, hematuria are helpful. Ultrasound abdomen is diagnostic of right-sided pyelonephritis.
3. *Perforated peptic ulcer:* History of dyspepsia may be present. Erect abdominal X-ray will reveal gas under diaphragm.
4. *Rectus sheath hematoma:* Mass may be palpable in the right iliac fossa, history of exercise will be present or the patient may be on anticoagulants. Ultrasound will help in diagnosing this condition.

Females

1. Right-sided salpingitis.
2. Tubo-ovarian mass.
3. *Mittelschmerz disease:* Midcycle rupture of a follicular cyst with bleeding produces lower abdominal and pelvic pain.
4. Torsion/hemorrhage of ovarian cyst.
5. *Ectopic pregnancy:* In unruptured tubal pregnancy, the pain remains on right side. Usually there is history of missed period, urinary pregnancy test is positive. Ruptured ectopic is an emergency.

LAPAROSCOPIC APPENDECTOMY (FIGS 10.3 TO 10.17A AND B)

Veress needle is introduced by making a small 1 cm incision in subumbilical region. Second port is in the right iliac fossa, which is a 10 mm port. This port is also used for retrieval of the appendix. Third port is in left iliac fossa and is 5 mm in diameter. Some surgeons put third port in suprapubic region in the midline, by doing this there is danger of injuring the bladder if it is full, and also by putting the port in left iliac fossa it is easy to handle the instrument. Retrieval of appendix[2] is done through the port in right iliac fossa if appendix is

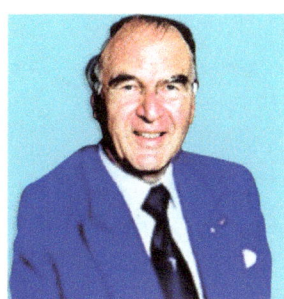

Fig. 10.3: Kurt Semm (1927–2003), Germany

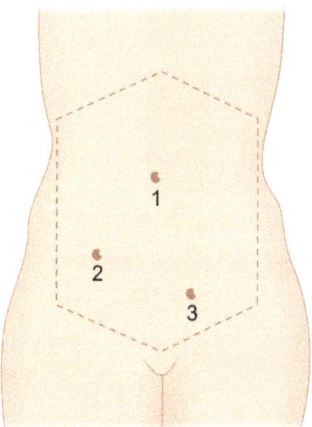

Fig. 10.4: Ports for laparoscopic appendectomy. 1, umbilical camera port; 2, 10 mm port in the right iliac fossa, right hand working port, (some surgeons introduce this port in the suprapubic region); 3, left hand working port in left iliac fossa.

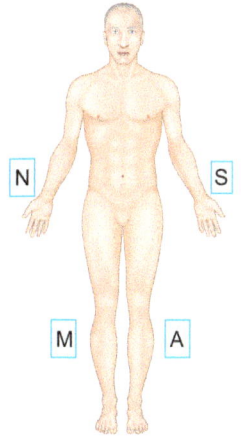

Fig. 10.5: Patient positioning. S, surgeon; A, assistant; N, nurse; M, monitor.

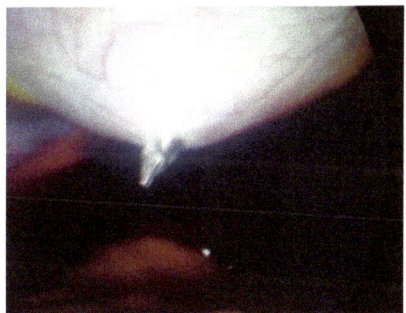

Fig. 10.6: Port entry under vision

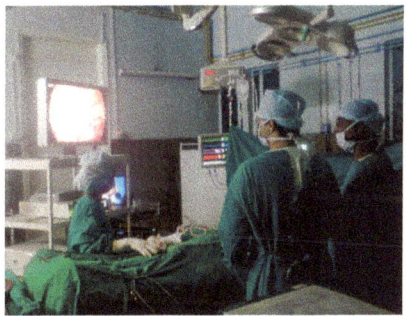

Fig. 10.7: Orientation of surgeon

64 Laparoscopic Appendectomy

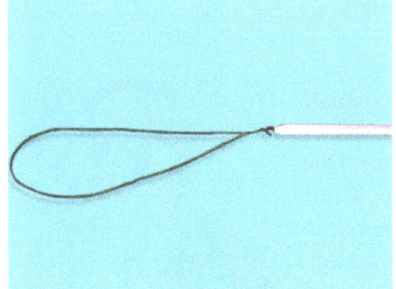

Fig. 10.8: Endoloop

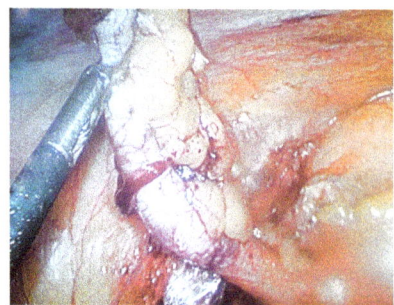

Fig. 10.9: Inflamed appendix

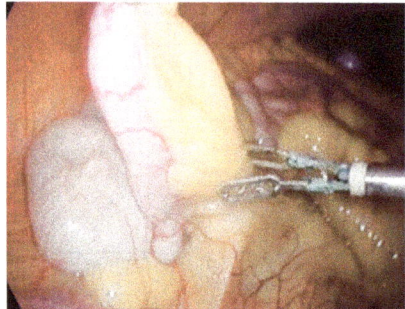

Fig. 10.10: Dissection of the mesoappendix

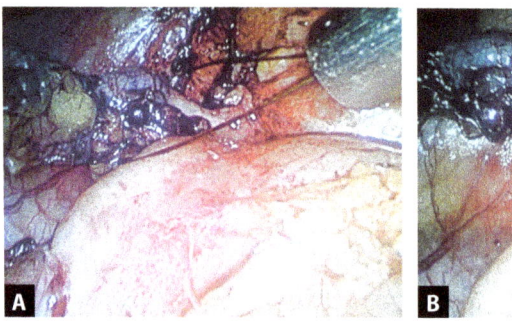

Figs 10.11A and B: Introducing the endoloop

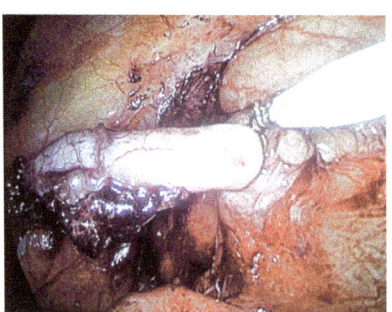

Fig. 10.12: Applying the endoloop

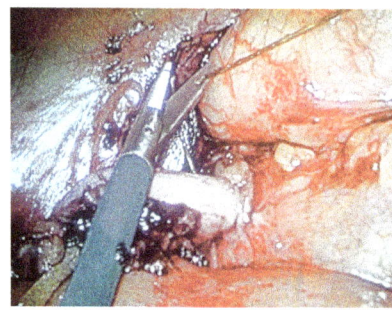

Fig. 10.13: Cutting using endoloop

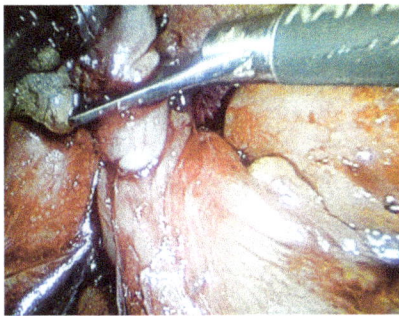

Fig. 10.14: Appendix being cut

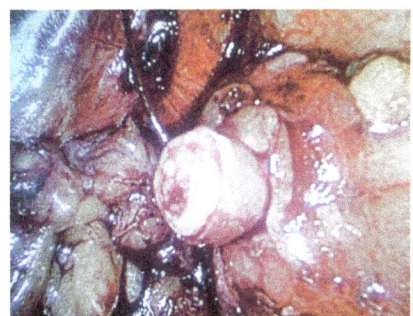

Fig. 10.15: Stump of the appendix

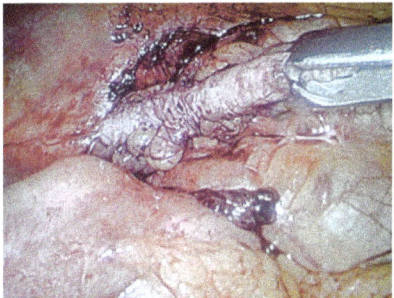

Fig. 10.16: Retrieval of specimen through 10 mm cannula

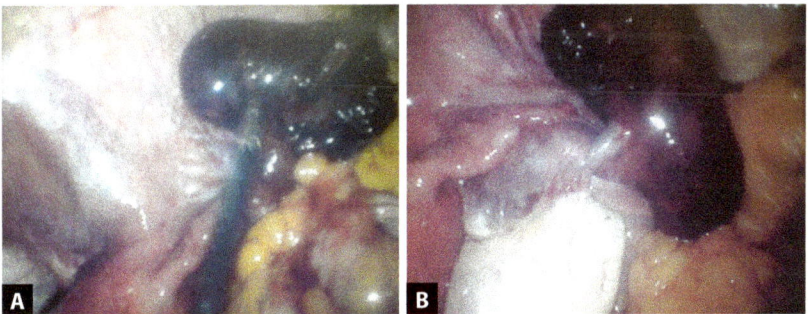

Figs 10.17A and B: Torsion of distal fallopian tube in a patient who hasundergone tubectomy

narrow and is removed in a bag if appendix is inflamed and bulky. Surgeon will be standing on the left of the patient, camera assistant on the left of the surgeon and monitor is placed on the right side of the patient towards foot end.

Laparoscopic appendectomy in rare anatomical positions is a better option than the big incisions needed for adequate access.[3] Laparoscopic appendectomy for complicated appendicitis is feasible and safe. It is associated with a significantly shorter operative time, lower incidence of wound infection and reduced length of hospital stay when compared to patients who had open appendectomy.[4]

REFERENCES

1. Bailey and Love's. Short Practice of Surgery, 25th edition. London: Edward Arnold Publishers Ltd; 2008.
2. Semm K. Endoscopic Appendectomy. Endoscopy. 1983;15(2):59-64.
3. C Palanivelu. Laparoscopic appendectomy for appendicitis in uncommon situations: the advantages of a tailored approach. Singapore Med J. 2007; 48(8):737.
4. Yau KK, Siu WT, Tang CN, et al. Laparoscopic versus open appendectomy for complicated appendicitis. J Am Coll Surg. 2007;205(1):60-5.

CHAPTER 11

Anatomy and Physiology of Gallbladder

SURGICAL ANATOMY OF GALLBLADDER

Gallbladder is a pear-shaped organ. The fundus is that portion, which projects from the free border of the liver. Fundus of the gallbladder is related to the angle formed by the lateral border of the rectus and the ninth coastal cartilage. When the fundus gets kinked upon itself it is known as Phrygian cap. Body of the gallbladder is the direct continuation of the fundus and constitutes the largest segment. The gallbladder body is attached to the visceral surface of the liver which is known as gallbladder bed.

This intimate relation of the gallbladder to the liver facilitates the direct spread of infection and neoplasm to the liver. The neck usually follows a gentle curve, the convexity of which may enlarge to form the infundibulum or Hartmann's pouch. It is attached to the duodenum through the cholecystoduodenal ligament. Outpouching of the inferior portion of the infundibulum is Hartmann's pouch.

Blood Supply

Cystic artery is a branch of right hepatic artery in 90% of the cases. It courses in the cystohepatic (Calot's triangle) triangle, which is bound by the cystic duct, hepatic duct and lower margin of liver.

Lymphatic Drainage

The lymphatics of the gallbladder (subserous and submucus) drain into the lymph node of lung. This lies in the fork created by the junction of cystic and common hepatic duct. The efferent vessels go the porta hepatic nodes and the celiac nodes. The subserous lymphatics communicate with the subcapsular lymphatics of the liver.

Anomalies of the Cystic Duct

Anomalies of the cystic duct (Figs 11.1A and B) have been described and are important during performance of cholecystectomy.[1] Cystic duct enters the common hepatic duct at an angle and the angle may vary from 80° to 10°. The cystic duct usually joins the common hepatic duct at an angle of 80°, but may run a parallel course with the common hepatic duct for a

Anatomy and Physiology of Gallbladder

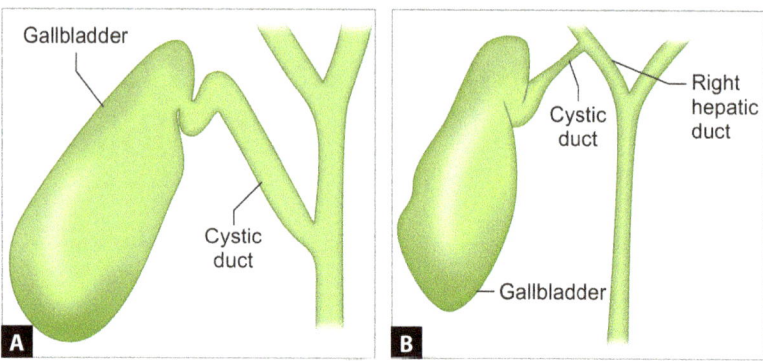

Figs 11.1A and B: Cystic duct. (A) Normal entry; (B) Cystic duct joining the right hepatic duct.

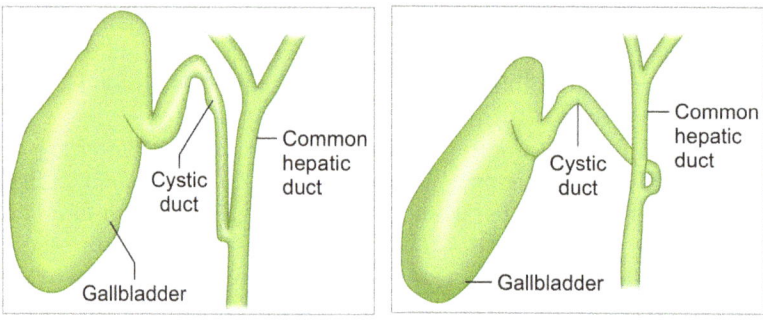

Fig. 11.2: Cystic duct parallel to the common hepatic duct

Fig. 11.3: Cystic duct posterior to the common hepatic duct

distance before joining it. In such case, the cystic duct is closely adherent to the common hepatic duct and effort to separate them will cause injury to the common hepatic duct. It is better to leave a long cystic duct stump in them. It may be dorsal to the duct and may join on its left side (spiral), which is present in 2% of the population. It may enter the right or left hepatic duct directly. The cystic duct may be short or absent in which case the gallbladder empties directly in the common hepatic duct.

Common hepatic duct (Figs 11.2 and 11.3) is formed by the union of the right and left hepatic ducts and is 2.5 cm long. Common bile duct is 7.5 cm long and is formed by the union of cystic duct to the common hepatic duct. It has four parts as given below:

1. The supraduodenal portion, about 2.5 cm long runs in the free border of lesser omentum.
2. The retroduodenal portion.
3. The infraduodenal portion, which lies in a tunnel on the posterior surface of the pancreas.
4. The intraduodenal portion passes through the wall of the second portion of the duodenum and is surrounded by the sphincter of oddi.

SURGICAL PHYSIOLOGY OF GALLBLADDER

Bile is composed of 97% of water, 1-2% of bile salts and 1% of pigments cholesterol and fatty acids. The liver excretes bile at the rate of 40 mL/hour. The primary bile salts cholate and chenodeoxycholate are synthesized in the liver from cholesterol. They are conjugated with taurine and glycine. Bile salts excreted in the bile help in digestion of fats.[2] In the intestine about 80% of the conjugated bile acids are absorbed in the terminal ileum. The remaining are deconjugated by the gut bacteria, forming secondary bile acids, deoxycholate and lithocholate. These are absorbed in the colon and transported back to the liver. This is enterohepatic circulation (95%). The remaining 5% gives the stool the color. The color of bile is due to the pigment bilirubin diglucuronide, which is derived by the breakdown of hemoglobin.[3]

Gallbladder Function

While fasting the resistance for the flow of bile through the sphincter of oddi is high therefore bile is diverted to the gallbladder after feeds the resistance is decreased and the bile enters the duodenum.

Main function of the gallbladder is active absorption of water, sodium chloride and bicarbonate by the mucus membrane. That is how low pressure is maintained in the biliary system. Gradual relaxation of the gallbladder and also emptying during fasting has a role to maintain low intraluminal pressure. The hepatic bile becomes concentrated 10 times in the gallbladder. Lastly it secretes about 20 mL of mucus per day.[4]

Neurohormonal Regulation

Hormonal receptors are located on the smooth muscles, vessels and epithelium of the gallbladder. Cholecystokinin (CCK) is a peptide secreted from the epithelium of the upper gastrointestinal tract and is found in highest concentration in the duodenum. It is released in the bloodstream by fats and amino acids.[5] It has a plasma half-life of 2-3 minutes. It contracts the gallbladder.[3] The vagus nerve stimulates contraction of the gallbladder and splanchnic sympathetic stimulation is inhibitory.

Sphincter of oddi: It acts as a high-pressure zone in between the duodenum and bile ducts. Normally, it regulates the flow of bile and pancreatic juice in the duodenum and prevents the regurgitation of duodenal contents in the biliary tree. It is a complex structure about 4-6 mm in length and has basal resting pressure of about 13 mm of mercury above the duodenal pressure. Relaxation occurs due to rise in CCK.

REFERENCES

1. Conlon K. Gallbladder and bile ducts. Bailey and Love's Short Practice of Surgery, 25th edition. Edward Arnold Publications Ltd; 2008. pp. 1111-29.

2. Boyer JL. Bile secretion models mechanism and malfunctions: A perspective on the development of modern cellular and molecular concepts of bile secretion and cholestasis. J Gastroenterol. 1996;31(3):475-81.
3. Oddsdottir M. Gallbladder and the extrahepatic biliary system. Schwartz's Principles of Surgery, 9th edition. McGraw-Hill Publishers; 2010. pp. 1137-39.
4. Benson E, et al. A practical reappraisal of the anatomy of the extrahepatic bile ducts and arteries. Br J Surg. 1976;63(11):853-60.
5. McDonnell CO, et al. The effect of cholecystectomy on plasma cholecystokinen. Am J of Gastroenterol. 2002;97(9):2189-92.

CHAPTER 12

Chronic Cholecystitis

NATURAL HISTORY

Most patients (80%) with gallstones remain asymptomatic throughout their life. They are diagnosed incidentally by ultrasonography or computed tomography (CT) scanning. Approximately, 2% of asymptomatic become symptomatic per year (biliary colic).[1] Once they become symptomatic then they tend to have recurrent bouts of biliary colic. Over a 20-year period over two third of gallstone individuals remain symptom free.[2]

Pure cholesterol stones account for less than 10% of the stones. They are single, large and have smooth surfaces. Most other cholesterol stones are usually multiple. They contain variable amount of pigments, but they must have more than 70% cholesterol by weight. Most of them are radiolucent. Cholesterol is insoluble in water. The primary event required for formation of stones is super saturation with cholesterol. Cholesterol solubility depends on the relative concentration of cholesterol, bile salts and lecithin (the main phospholipid in bile). Super saturation always occur because of the increased secretion of cholesterol rather than under secretion of bile salts and lecithin.[3] Pigment stones contain less than 30% cholesterol and are dark, because of presence of calcium bilirubinate.

Chronic Cholecystitis (Biliary Colic)

About two-thirds of patients of symptomatic gallstones present with chronic cholecystitis. Chronic cholecystitis is characterized by recurrent attacks of right upper quadrant or epigastric pain, which usually follows heavy meals.[4] The pain radiates around the sides to the tip of the right scapula. Sometimes it radiates straight through the back. Nausea and vomiting may occur during an attack of colic. Self-induced vomiting makes the patient comfortable. Pain is episodic and the intervals between the episodes are variable. Bloating and belching may be present in between the attacks. Physical findings are present only during the attack. These include right upper quadrant or epigastric tenderness and muscle guarding. The gallbladder is not palpable.

The pain occurs due to temporary obstruction of the gallbladder outlet. The pain follows heavy meals as there is release of cholecystokinin, which causes gallbladder contraction.

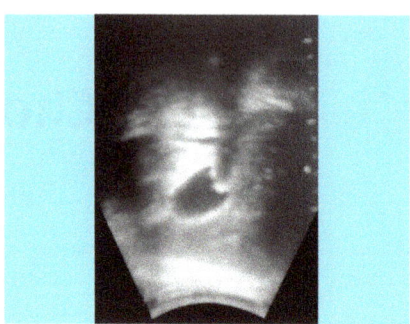

Fig. 12.1: Acoustic shadowing of the gallstone

The diagnosis is confirmed by ultrasonography, which has got a 98% sensitivity and specificity.[5] Stones produce acoustic shadow (Fig. 12.1). The other important criteria is the stones move with the change in position of the patient. The advantages with ultrasonography are that it is noninvasive, no preparation is required, easily available, no radiation, cost effective and is safe.

Porcelain Gallbladder

Deposition of calcium on the chronically inflamed gallbladder results in porcelain gallbladder. The calcific outline can be seen on the plain films. The presence of porcelain gallbladder is an indication for cholecystectomy as it is a premalignant condition. The gallbladder will be contracted with dense adhesions scarring and fibrosis are present.

REFERENCES

1. Gracie WA, et al. The natural history of silent gallstones; the innocent gallstone is not a myth. N Eng J Med. 1982;307(13):798-800.
2. Attilii AF, et al. The natural history of gallstones. The GREPCO experience. Hepatology. 1995;21(3):655-60.
3. Klein AS, et al. Liver biliary tract and pancreas, physiologic basis of surgery. Baltimore: Williams & Wilkins; 1996. p. 441.
4. Oddsdottir M. Gallbladder and the extrahepatic biliary system. Schwartz's Principles of Surgery, 9th edition. McGraw-Hill Publishers; 2010. pp. 1145-6.
5. Cooperberg PL, et al. Real time ultrasonography. Diagnostic treatment of choice in calculus gallbladder disease. N Eng J Med. 1980;302(23):1277-9.

CHAPTER 13

Acute Cholecystitis

The primary event that needs to occur in acute cholecystitis is obstruction of the cystic duct. This obstruction leads to distension of the gallbladder, subserous edema and inflammation of the wall (Fig. 13.1). The wall becomes grossly thickened and subserous hemorrhages occur and pericholecystic fluid is present. The mucosa becomes hyperemic. Secondary bacterial infection occurs in 30% of the patients and this may give rise to empyema. Rarely necrosis of the wall may lead to perforation, and more frequently the stone may get dislodged and the inflammation subsides.[1] Perforation may give rise to localized abscess, intrahepatic abscess peritonitis or cholecystoenteric fistula.

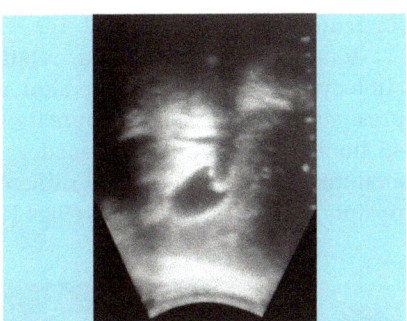

Fig. 13.1: Stone in the gallbladder with acoustic shadow

CLINICAL FEATURES

About 80% of the patients have a prior history of chronic cholecystitis. Acute cholecystitis starts as biliary colic, but the pain unremitting. The pain is present in the right upper quadrant or epigastric region and radiates to the back. Nausea, vomiting, fever and guarding, which obscures the mass are present. On examination, tenderness and rigidity are present in the right hypochondrium.

Murphy's Sign

The inspiratory arrest on deep palpation in the right hypochondrium is characteristic. Mild-to-moderate leukocytosis is present.

Ultrasonography

Ultrasonography has a sensitivity and specificity of 95%. It will also detect thickening and pericholecystic collection.

Tenderness in the gallbladder area by probe is sonologic Murphy's sign. It will also demonstrate the dilation of the common bile duct and there will be leukocytosis.

TREATMENT

Patients who present with cholecystitis require IV fluids, antibiotics and analgesics.[2] The antibiotics should cover gram-negative aerobes and anaerobes. For patients who have allergies for cephalosporin, aminoglycoside with metronidazole may be given. Cholecystectomy is the definitive treatment for acute cholecytitis.[3]

Acute cholecystitis is a relative contraindication for laparoscopic cholecystectomy. The conversion rate is higher (10-15%). If the patient presents more than 48-72 hours then the technical difficulty increases. After 48 hours, the edema, increased vascularity and distortion of the normal anatomy will pose technical difficulties. In such case, the surgery may be postponed to after 6-8 weeks (Figs 13.2 to 13.6).

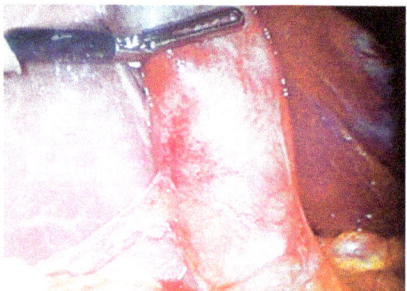

Fig. 13.2: Holding at the fundus

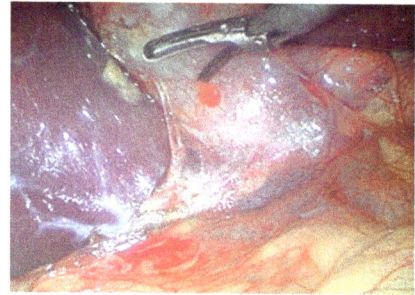

Fig. 13.3: Adhesions being released

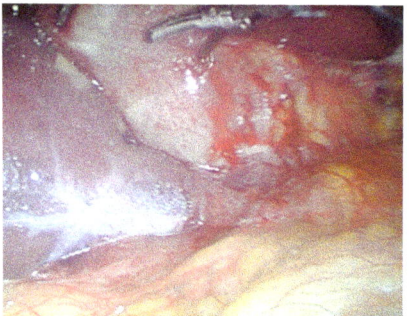

Fig. 13.4: Dissection continued

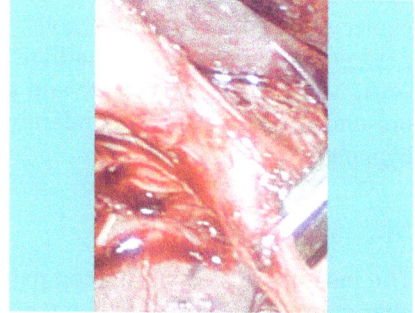

Fig. 13.5: Cystic duct being isolated

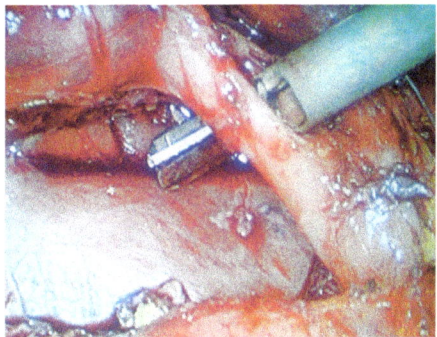

Fig. 13.6: Cystic duct identified

ACALCULOUS CHOLECYSTITIS

Inflammation of the gallbladder without the gallstones is said to be acalculous cholecystitis. This usually occurs in ill patients of the intensive care unit. Patients on parenteral nutrition, extensive burns and sepsis, and major operations are candidates for acalculous cholecystitis.

REFERENCES

1. Strasberg SM. Cholelithiasis and acute cholecystitis. Baillieres Clin Gastroenterol. 1997;11(4):643-61.
2. Margaret oddsdottir. Schwartz principles of surgery, 9th edition. Gallbladder and the Extrahepatic Biliary System. McGraw-Hill Publishers; 2010. pp. 1147-8.
3. Kiviluoto T, Sirén J, Luukkonen P, et al. Randomised trial of laparoscopic versus open cholecystectomy for acute and gangrenous cholecystitis. Lancet. 1998 31;351(9099):321-5.

CHAPTER 14

Laparoscopic Cholecystectomy

■ HISTORY OF CHOLECYSTECTOMY

In the late 1980s, laparoscopy was essentially a gynecologist's tool. One of the French private surgeons, Philippe Mouret of Lyon, shared his surgery practice with a gynecologist, and thus had access to both laparoscopic equipment and to patients requiring laparoscopy. In March 1987, Mouret carried out his first cholecystectomy by means of electronic laparoscopy.[1] Although he never published anything about this experience, the news on his technique reached Francois Dubois of Paris. Without any prior laparoscopic experience, Dubois acted immediately. He borrowed the instruments from gynecologists, performed his first animal experiments and, in April 1988, carried out the first laparoscopic cholecystectomy in Paris. Inspired by Dubois, Jacques Perissat of Bordeaux, introduced endoscopic cholecystectomy in his clinic and presented this technique at a Society of American Gastrointestinal Surgeons (SAGES) meeting in Louisville, in April 1989.[2] Very soon, news of the French work in LC soon swept beyond the country's borders. Dubois and Perissat spoke enthusiastically about their work at the meetings and were largely responsible for establishing what is today called the French technique.[3]

It was not until after 1986, following the development of a video computer chip that allowed the magnification and projection of images onto television screens that the techniques of laparoscopic surgery truly became integrated into the discipline of general surgery. The first laparoscopic cholecystectomy performed on a human patient was done in 1987 by the French physician Mouret. The rapid acceptance of the technique of laparoscopic surgery by the general population is unparalleled in surgical history. It has changed the field of general surgery more drastically and more rapidly than any other surgical milestone.[4] In 1882, Carl Langebuch (1846-1901) of Germany performed the first cholecystectomy.[4] In 1985, Erich Mühe, a professor of surgery in Boblingen, Germany, used Semm's instruments and technique to remove the first gallbladder in the world laparoscopically. Three years later, when Semm presented a videotape of his laparoscopic appendectomy in Baltimore, he gave impetus to Barry McKernan J (general surgeon) and William B. Saye (gynecologist) of Marietta, Georgia, to carry out the first laparoscopic cholecystectomy in the United States.

Shortly thereafter the 'laparoscopic revolution' broke out and Semm's laparoscopic expertise was in great demand. His publications on the subject, translated into many languages, were read across the world by thousands of surgeons. Without Semm's input, the development of a 'laparoscopic revolution', while perhaps inevitable, would have been postponed by many years. Medicine made a tremendous leap forward. The German Surgical Society rejected Mühe in 1986 after he reported that he had performed the first laparoscopic cholecystectomy, yet in 1992 he received their highest award, the German Surgical Society Anniversary Award.

In 1990, in Atlanta, at the SAGES Convention, Perissat, Berci, Cuschieri, Dubois and Mouret were recognized by SAGES for performing early laparoscopic cholecystectomies, but Mühe was not. However, in 1999 he was recognized by SAGES for having performed the first laparoscopic cholecystectomy and invited Mühe to present the Storz lecture. In Mühe's presentation titled 'The First Laparoscopic Cholecystectomy,' which he gave in March 1999 in San Antonio, Texas, he described the first procedure. Finally, Mühe had received the worldwide acclaim that he deserved for his pioneering work.[4, 5]

OPERATIVE SETUP

Laparoscopic cholecystectomy is done under general anesthesia. The patient has to be strapped securely as the tilts in the table may risk the patient to fall. Ryles tube is routinely introduced in the cases and is removed the next day on the rounds. As this helps in the deflation of the stomach. Distended stomach and duodenum greatly obscure the field. The head end of the table is tilted upwards, this will make the liver fall downwards. Right side of the patient is tilted upwards. Surgeon stands on the left side of the patient, on the left side of the surgeon is camera assistant. On the right side of the patient is second assistant retracting the fundus of gallbladder. Monitor is at the right side at the head end of patient (Fig. 14.1).

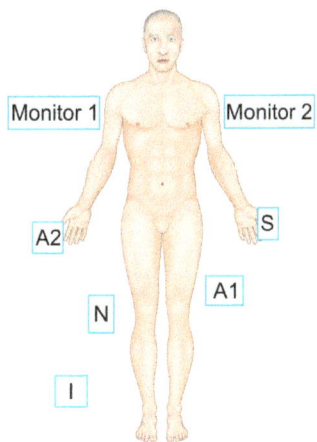

Fig. 14.1: Patient positioning in laparoscopic cholecystectomy. S, surgeon; A1, assistant 1; A2, assistant 2; N, nurse;I, instrument table.

PORT POSITIONS (Fig. 14.2)

First Port

The first port is the infraumbilical port for the camera, second 10 mm port is the epigastric port for the surgeons right hand. Third port is the right midclavicular port for the surgeon's left hand. Fourth port is the right anterior axillary port for the retraction of the fundus towards the right shoulder of the patient (Fig. 14.3).

Laparoscopic Cholecystectomy

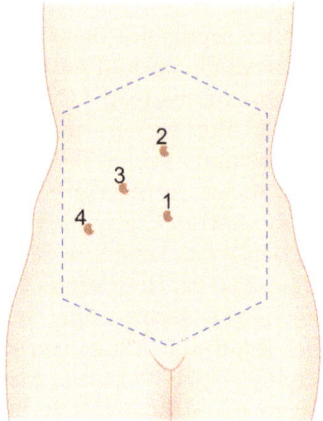

Fig. 14.2: Port position. 1. Umbilical port; 2. Epigastric port; 3. Right midclavicular port; 4. Anterior axillary port.

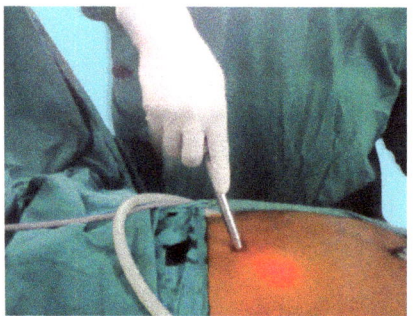

Fig. 14.3: Epigastric port being introduced with the camera inside (external view)

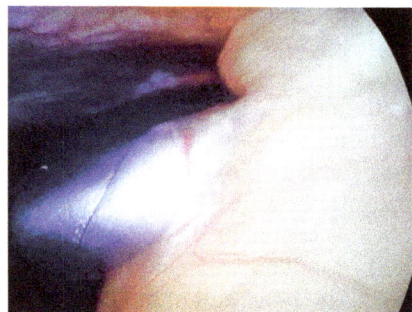

Fig. 14.4: Epigastric port entering to the right of the falciform ligament

Second Port

Second port trocar is inserted just right of falciform ligament. 10 mm epigastric port is introduced as high as possible, as this will help in identifying the tip of the right hand instrument easily. This is important because viewing both the jaws of clip applicator is important. The angle between the camera and the right hand instrument should be >90º (Fig. 14.4).

Third Port

A 5 mm port is in the right midclavicular line just below the coastal margin, a grasping forceps introduced through this trocar will hold the Hartmann's pouch, and apply gentle downward and lateral traction. This maneuver will help in the opening of the Calot's triangle (Fig. 14.5).

If too much traction is applied on the left hand then there may be tenting of the common bile duct (CBD) giving rise to serious injury (transection) to the CBD. The dissection should be carried out on either side of the infundibulum. The peritoneum on the lateral side of the infundibulum is dissected.

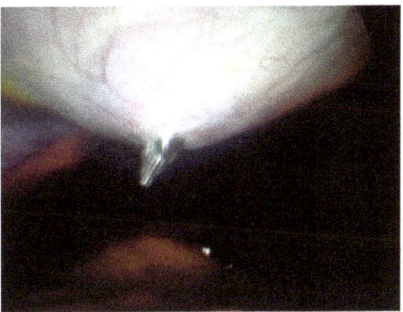

Fig. 14.5: Midclavicular port being inserted

Fourth Port

Fourth port is a 5 mm port and is in the anterior axillary line again below the coastal margin. Grasping forceps with ratchet is introduced through this port to hold the fundus and retracted towards the right shoulder of the patient. Sometimes when the gallbladder wall is thick or if there is edema of the gallbladder, it is difficult to hold the fundus with the grasper in such a situation the option available is to change the trocar to 10 mm and hold the fundus of the gallbladder with a crocodile forceps, in order to retract it. If the liver is cirrhotic then the mobility is restricted (Fig. 14.6).

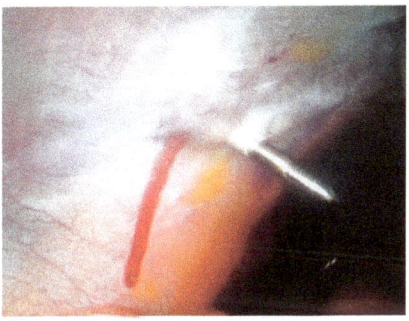

Fig. 14.6: Fourth port being inserted In the right anterior axillary line

■ PROCEDURE

Initial Dissection

The fundus of the gallbladder is held with a grasper (with ratchet) and retracted towards the right shoulder of the patient, this also lifts the right lobe of the liver and exposes the Calot's triangle. Adhesions on the under surface of the gallbladder are released beginning from the fundus and proceeding downwards. Adhesions are held in the left hand and retracted downwards they may contain the omentum, colon, stomach and duodenum (Figs 14.7 to 14.12A and B).

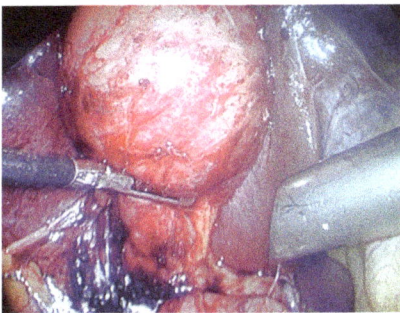

Fig. 14.7: Identifying fundus of gallbladder

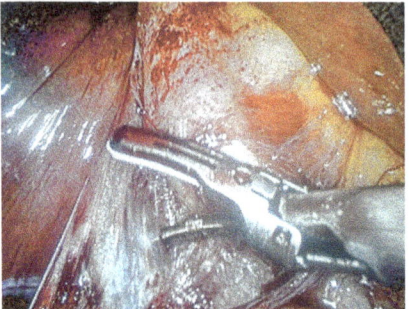

Fig. 14.8: Adhesions to the gallbladder being released

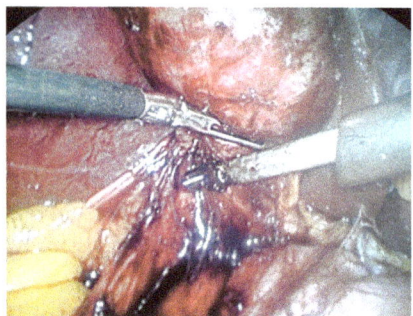

Fig. 14.9: Dissection continued

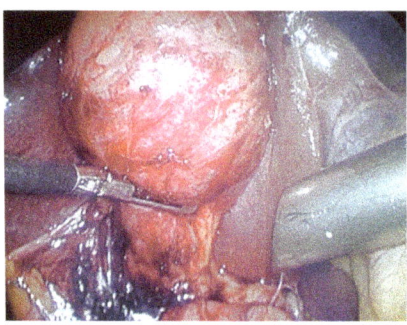

Fig. 14.10: Mucocele of gallbladder: Omental adhesions being released

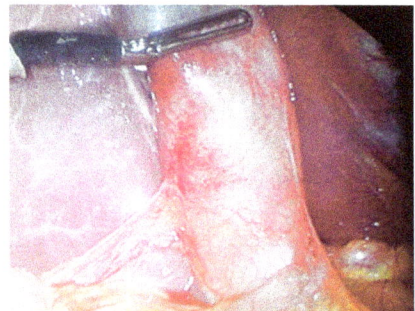

Fig. 14.11: Adhesions in acute cholecystitis

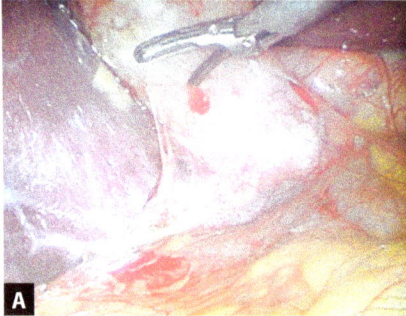
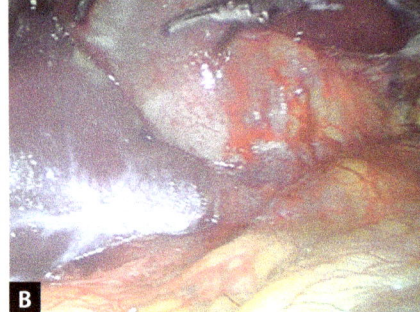

Figs 14.12A and B: Omental adhesions being released

A grossly distended gallbladder is difficult to grasp without the risk of rupture, in such a situation it has to be aspirated with a spinal needle attached to a syringe inserted through the abdomen under vision. Bile leak from the puncture site can be prevented by grasping the fundus at this site.

A thick gallbladder requires a toothed grasper for retraction. In some conditions, the liver is adherent to the anterior abdominal wall in which condition it is difficult to retract it. In fibrotic cirrhotic liver there is portal hypertension leading to increased bleeding.

Dissection of the Calot's Triangle

Triangle of Calot is defined by the cystic duct, common hepatic duct and the lower edge of the liver. Too vigorous dissection in this triangle will lead to bleeding. To prevent this, the initial dissection is started on the lateral aspect of the Calot's triangle, dividing the lateral peritoneal attachment of the infundibulum from the liver allows mobilization of the infundibulum. Dissection on the lateral aspect of the infundibum allows identification of the lateral margin of cystic duct, the dissection is then carried on the medial aspect (Figs 14.13 and 14.14).

Once the infundibulum is free, it is held with the left hand and retracted outwards and to the right of the patient. The anterior aspect of the Calot's triangle is exposed.

The dissection is begun on the infundibulum of the gallbladder, using a harmonic scalpel and peritoneum is dissected both on the anterior and posterior aspects. Moving of the left hand infundibular grasper inferolaterally and superomedially will help in this dissection.

Identification and Clip Application of Cystic Duct and Artery

Using a right-angled forceps a window is created posterior to the cystic duct, also the joining of the cystic duct, to the common hepatic duct is identified. The cystic duct and the cystic artery are skeletanized.

Two clips are applied on the cystic duct towards the CBD and one clip towards the specimen. Same is done for the cystic artery. The duct and the artery are cut (Figs 14.15 to 14.25).

Dissection from the Liver Bed

The liver is retracted upwards so that the gallbladder bed is visualized always. The instrument that we routinely used for mobilizing of the gallbladder from

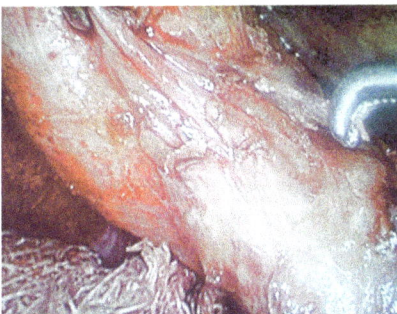

Fig. 14.13: Lymph node dissection in the Calot's triangle

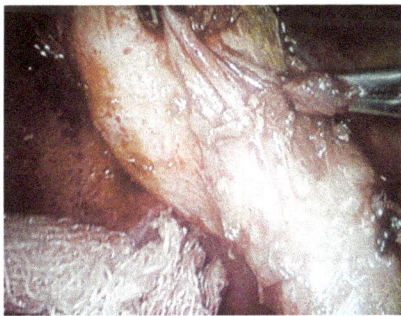

Fig. 14.14: Lymph node in the Calot's triangle isolated

Laparoscopic Cholecystectomy

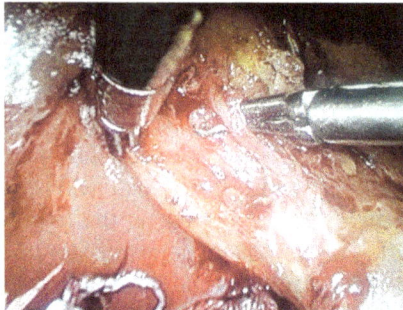

Fig. 14.15: Cystic artery isolation with the help of right-angled forceps

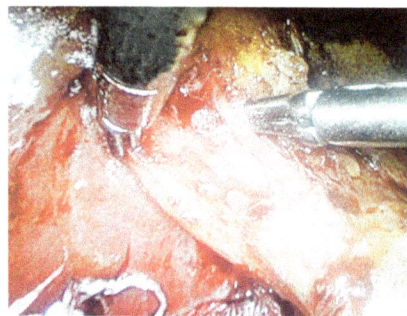

Fig. 14.16: Cystic artery being isolated

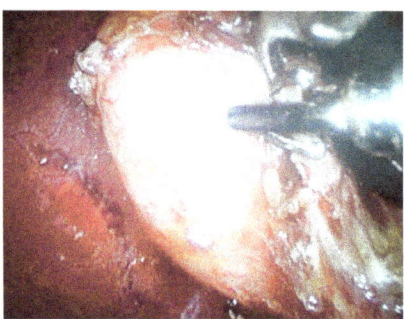

Fig. 14.17: Clips being applied on cystic artery

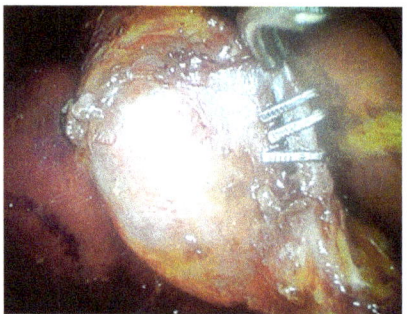

Fig. 14.18: Three clips applied on the cystic artery

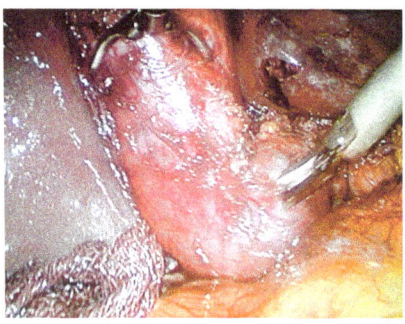

Fig. 14.19: Neck of the gallbladder

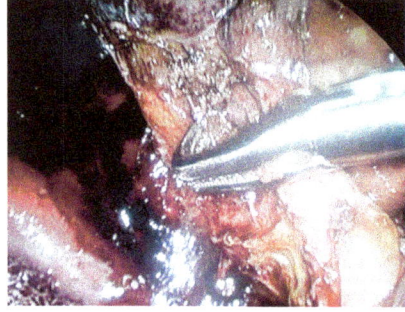

Fig. 14.20: Posterior dissection

the liver bed is spatula with monopolar cautery. The surgeon's left hand pulling the infundibulum laterally acts as traction, the assistants grasper holding the fundus and retracting towards the right shoulder of the patient acts as counter traction. In an uninflamed gallbladder, the plane between the gallbladder and the liver is avascular whereas in chronically inflamed gallbladder, it may be densely adherent to the liver and may bleed. There is possibility of entering the liver tissue at a deeper plane giving rise to bleeding

Laparoscopic Cholecystectomy

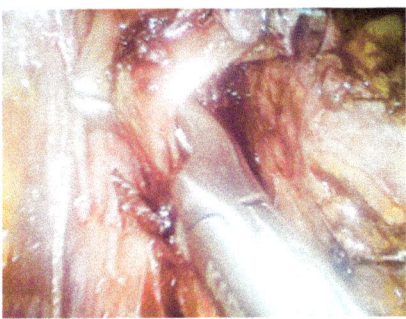

Fig. 14.21: Cystic duct being isolated

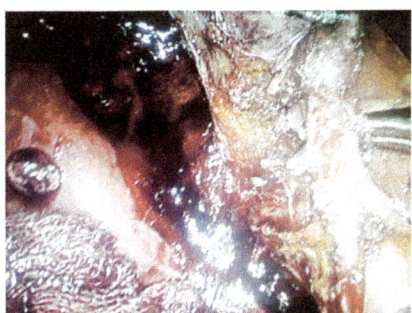

Fig. 14.22: Right-angled forceps dissecting the cystic duct window being created.

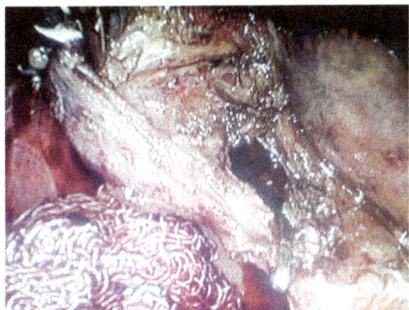

Fig. 14.23: One clip applied on the cystic duct

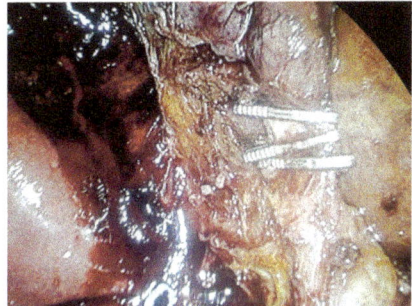

Fig. 14.24: Three clips applied on the cystic duct

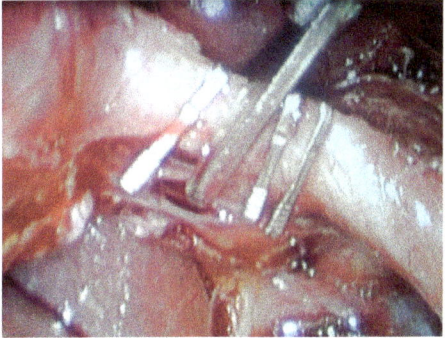

Fig. 14.25: Cystic duct being cut between two clips applied towards the common bile duct and one towards the gallbladder

or if the gallbladder is very thin there may be rupture of the wall giving rise to bile leak, in this situation the rent can be closed using a clip or endoloop. Fundal dissection from the bed is left incomplete to use the gallbladder for traction. The clips applied to the cystic duct and the arteries are visualized after cleaning the abdominal cavity by irrigation and suction. Then fundal

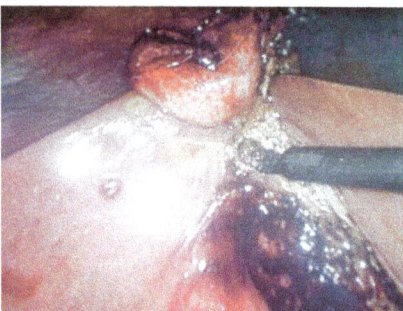 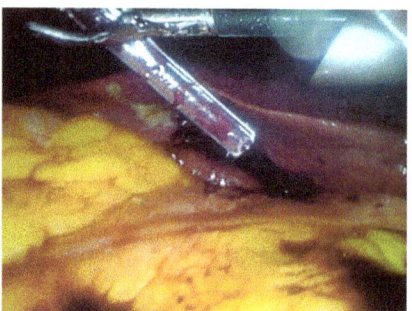

Fig. 14.26: Gallbladder being dissected from the bed

Fig. 14.27: Drain being introduced from the right anterior axillary port

dissection is completed. Before dividing the final attachments of the gallbladder, the gallbladder bed should be inspected for bleeding and leak of bile from duct of Luschka also the clips on the cystic artery and the duct are inspected to ensure that they are not dislodged during mobilization. Once the gallbladder is completely separated from the liver bed, the liver will fall down to its normal position, and the inspection of cystic artery and duct will become difficult after the gallbladder is detached, it is kept over the liver (Fig. 14.26).

Drain

Routinely, suction (romovac) drain is placed through the anterior axillary port. The valve of the cannula is removed and drain is inserted through the cannula with a artery forceps applied to the drain in order to prevent the gas leak, Allis forceps is applied to the drain externally along with the skin (Fig. 14.27).

Extraction of the Gallbladder

Routinely, bag is used for removal of the gallbladder as this reduces the possibility of infection of the port site. The bag edges are cut differentially so that the separation of the edges becomes easier within the abdomen. Any clots or the spilled stones can be introduced in the bag. The grasper holding the bag along with the trocar is removed through the abdominal wall as single unit under vision. Once the opening of the bag has come into view, it is held with external artery forceps and the mouth of the bag is opened widely, the gallbladder is cut open to suck the bile. During this procedure the camera assistant keeps gallbladder under vision. A hemostat can be passed by the side of the bag through the epigastric port and the jaws opened gently to dilate the fascia, permitting easier extraction of the bag at no point should undue force applied for extraction as the bag may give way at the lower end and the specimen may fall in the peritoneal cavity (Figs 14.28 to 14.33).

Laparoscopic Cholecystectomy

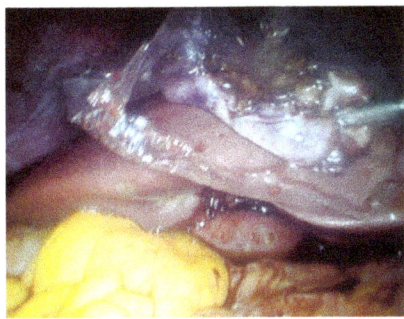

Fig. 14.28: Gallbladder being introduced in the bag

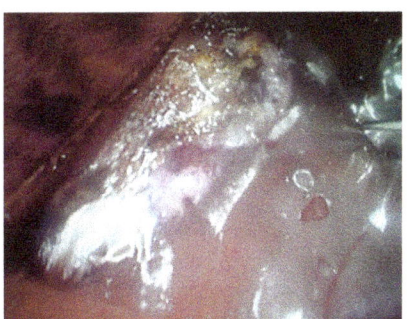

Fig. 14.29: Plastic bag being withdrawn from the peritoneal cavity

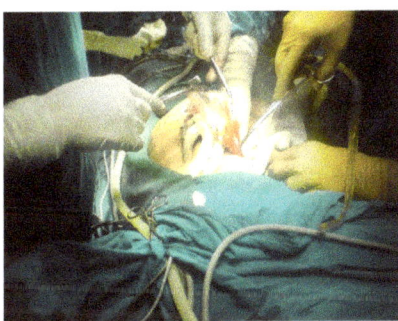

Fig. 14.30: Extraction of the gallbladder in a bag (external view)

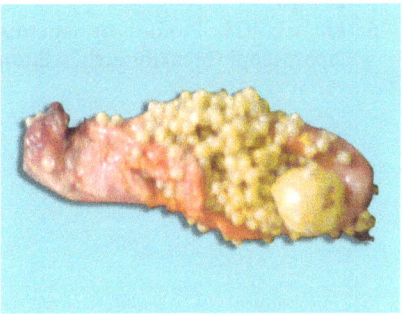

Fig. 14.31: Specimen of gallbladder studded with stones

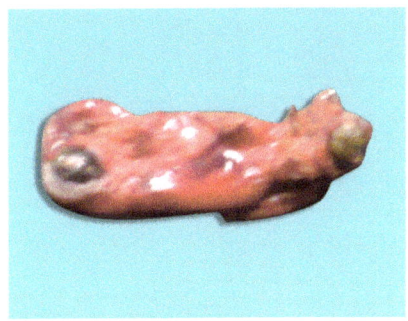

Fig. 14.32: Gallbladder with two stones: One in the body and other in the Hartmann's pouch

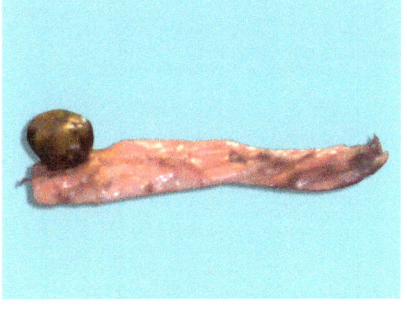

Fig. 14.33: Large-sized solitary stone of the gallbladder

Floppy Left Lobe of Liver

Sometimes, the left lobe of the liver is very floppy and falls in the operative field obscuring the vision. Using the angled scope will not solve the problem.

To overcome the problem the liver has to be torqued. The fundus of the gallbladder has to be lifted upward and medially. This will cause rotation of the liver on its axis. This will allow the left lobe to fall away.

REFERENCES

1. Walker Reynolds Jr. The First Laparoscopic Cholecystectomy. JSLS. 2001; 5(1):89-94.
2. Bruce v Macfadeyen. Laparoscopic surgery of the abdomen. Laparoscopic cholecystectomy. New York: Springer-Verlag; 2004. pp. 71-86.
3. Spaner SJ, Warnock GL. A brief history of endoscopy, laparoscopy, and laparoscopic surgery. J Laparoendosc Adv Surg Tech A. 1997;7(6):369-73.
4. Litynski GS. The American Spirit Awakens. In: Litynski GS (Ed). Highlights in the History of Laparoscopy. Frankfurt, Germany: Barbara Bernert Verlag; 1996. pp. 227-70.
5. Litynski GS. Profiles in laparoscopy: Mouret, Dubois, and Perissat: the laparoscopic breakthrough in Europe (1987-1988). JSLS. 1999;3(2):163-7.

CHAPTER 15

Diagnostic Laparoscopy

PROCEDURE

Umbilicus represents the thinnest part of the abdominal wall where the fascia and the skin are tethered together. This is the site chosen for the insertion of the Veress needle. The alternative site is the Palmer's point, i.e. 2 cm below the left coastal margin and the enlarged spleen is at risk at this point.

The umbilical port is used for laparoscope. If right lower quadrant pain is a indication then the second port is introduced either in the midline suprapubically or in the left lower quadrant. This allows manipulation of the bowel (Fig. 15.1) and pelvic organs. If upper abdomen is the presenting problem then left upper quadrant port with possible addition of the epigastric port is considered for the manipulation of upper abdominal organs. The second puncture is made under laparoscopic guidance after infiltration with 2% lignocaine in the preperitoneum.[1] The surgeon should stand opposite the area being exposed.

INDICATIONS

- Acute abdominal pain
- Chronic abdominal pain
- Trauma
- Liver tumors
- Liver disease
- Ascites
- Infertility
- Tumor staging
- Mass abdomen
- Miscellaneous.

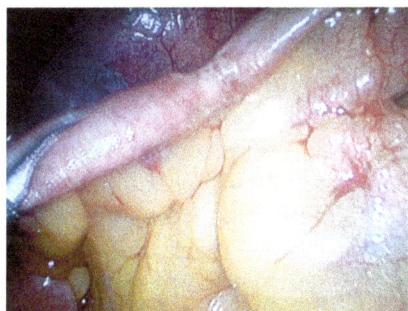

Fig. 15.1: Bowel being 'run' through in diagnostic laparoscopy

Acute Abdomen

Acute lower abdominal pain in females is ideal for laparoscopy.[2] The various causes encountered in acute abdomen are appendicitis, terminal ileitis, mesenteric adenitis, Meckel's diverticulitis, salpingitis (Fig. 15.2), pelvic inflammatory disease, adnexal torsion and ectopic pregnancy, ruptured ovarian cyst.[3]

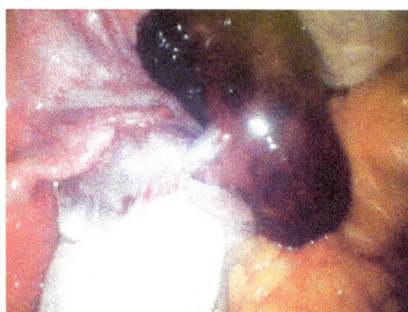

Fig. 15.2: Torsion of the right distal salpinx following tubectomy

Ruptured Corpus Luteal Cyst

There will be remnants of the cyst on the ovary along with presence of fluid in the pelvis. A hemorrhagic cyst will show evidence of hemorrhage. The condition is associated with the absence of other pathology. Irrigation of the pelvis alone is required.

Ectopic Pregnancy

Tubal pregnancy often appears as a bulge in the tube with a bluish hue.[4] Salpingectomy or salpingostomy need to be done. The treatment depends on the patient's desire to maintain fertility, the condition of the tube.

In case of abdominal mass, when the non-invasive methods fail to accurately localize then diagnostic laparoscopy can be done with biopsy.

Chronic Abdominal/Pelvic Pain

Chronic pelvic pain is defined as pain below the line joining the two anterior superior iliac spines for more than 6 months, causing functional disability and requiring treatment.[5] Patients with chronic pelvic pain are frequently depressed, anguished and distressed. The various causes of chronic pelvic pain are pelvic inflammatory disease, endometriosis and adhesions. This study concludes that diagnostic laparoscopy is gold standard in the evaluation of chronic pelvic pain.

Infertility

Diagnostic laparoscopy has been included as a standard work-up procedure in infertility. The fimbria, tubes, uterus and ovaries can be evaluated. The patency of the fallopian tubes can be assessed by chromotubation. The failure of the dye to pass freely indicates intramural pathology.

Liver Disease

In liver disease, when standard biopsy fails then diagnostic laparoscopy with liver biopsy is indicated.[6]

Liver Tumors

More than 75% of the liver surface can be visualized during laparoscopy. About 80-90% of the primary and secondary liver malignancies are on the surface. Biopsy can be done.

Peritoneal Tuberculosis

More than 40% do not involve the alimentary tract and are present in bizarre manner.[7]

Ascitic Form

The peritoneum is studded with tubercles (Fig. 15.3) and there is ascites. The ascitic fluid is rich in lymphocyte. Weakness, pallor and loss of weight are present. Pain abdomen may be present. On palpation an indistinct mass may be palpated, which is rolled up omentum.

Encysted Form

Encysted form is similar to the ascetic form, but is localized to a particular region. In case of children, the swelling is difficult to distinguish from mesenteric cyst. The collection has to be evacuated and cyst wall excised and sent for histopathology.

Fibrous Form

In fibrous form, the coils of intestine become adherent to one another. These distended coils act as blind loops and give rise to pain abdomen wasting and steatorrhea.

Purulent Form

Purulent form is rare, cold abscess present in between the coils of intestine.

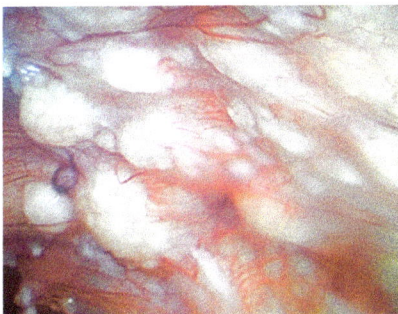

Fig. 15.3: Tubercular abdomen (nodules on the peritoneum)

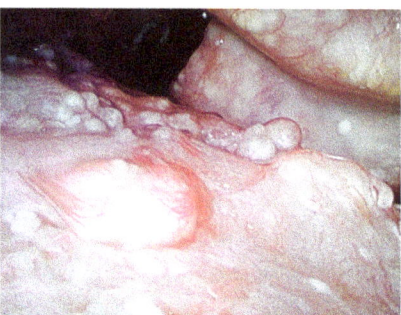

Fig. 15.4: Abdominal tuberculosis

Intestinal Tuberculosis

Tuberculosis can affect any part of the gastrointestinal tract from the oral cavity to the anus (Fig. 15.4).[8] The most commonly affected site is the ileocecal region, because of the ileocecal valve, long contact period and stasis of intestinal contents in this region.

Hypertrophic Ileocecal Tuberculosis

The hypertrophic ileocecal tuberculosis is caused by ingestion of *Mycobacterium tuberculosis* in people who have good resistance. The infection establishes in the lymphoid follicles. There is thickening of the intestinal wall and narrowing of the lumen. They usually present with pain abdomen, loss of weight is present and on examination there may be a mass in the right iliac fossa.

Ulcerative Ileocecal Tuberculosis

Ulcerative ileocecal tuberculosis is secondary to pulmonary tuberculosis and occurs due to swallowing of tubercle bacilli. There are multiple ulcers in the terminal ileum which are placed transversely. The overlying serosa is red.

Barium meal follow-through or small bowel enema will show absence of filling of the terminal ileum, cecum and ascending colon due to hypermotility and narrowing.

Tuberculous Mesenteric Lymphadenitis

Tuberculous mesenteric lymphadenitis is less common than non-specific lymphadenitis. Tubercle bacilli (bovine) are ingested and enter the mesenteric nodes through the Peyer's patches. Children are the victims. They present with pain abdomen.

Adhesiolysis

Adhesions are the most common cause of small bowel obstruction. In most patients adhesions do not cause any problem, but in some cases there will be adhesion-related disease. Intra-abdominal adhesions are one of the common problems encountered during laparoscopic surgery (Figs 15.5A to G).

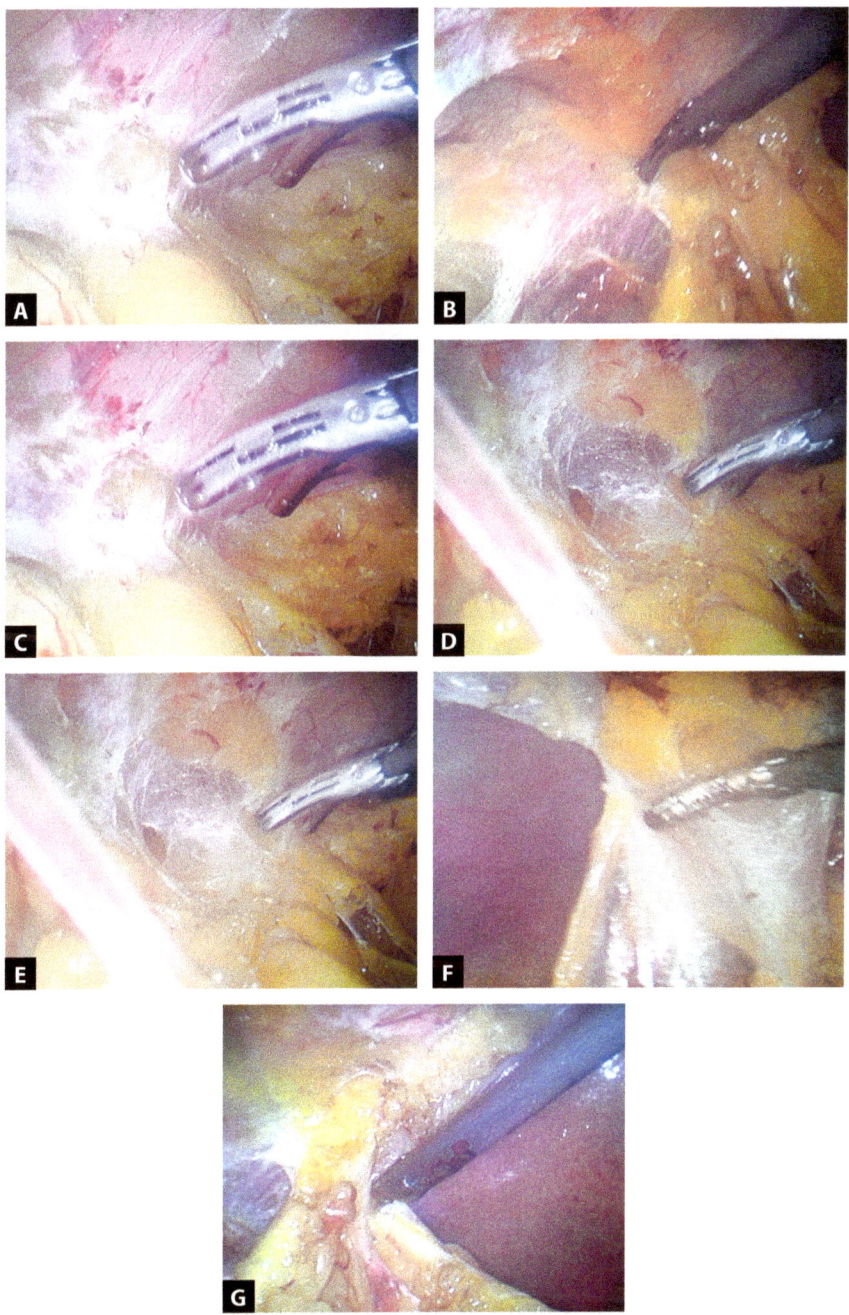

Figs 15.5A to G: Releasing adhesions between the anterior abdominal wall and bowel

Access

Initial port entry should be far away from the abdominal scar. The commonly chosen point is the Palmer's point, which is in the left midclavicular line below the costal margin. Some surgeons follow the open method of entry. The principles that required to be followed are:
1. Angled scope should be used so that the view becomes easier.
2. The adhesions should be stretched and opened up to visualize the anatomy.
3. The adhesions are least vascular at the point of attachment to the anterior abdominal wall rather than at the center of the fibrous band.

Trauma

A prerequisite for the use of diagnostic laparoscopy in the management of abdominal trauma is that the patient should be hemodynamically stable.[1] Superficial liver lacerations constitute more than 50% of the liver injuries and stop bleeding spontaneously requiring no treatment.[9] Blunt injury to the abdomen is far more common than penetrating injury.[10] Out of 1083 patients admitted for trauma only 138 were penetrating injuries in a Taiwanese study group. Laparoscopy for evaluating blunt trauma is less evaluated than for assessing penetrating trauma.[11]

In penetrating trauma about 30–50% of the stab wounds does not penetrate the peritoneum and another 20–40% with peritoneal penetration do not involve significant injuries, resulting in no-therapeutic laparotomies.[12,13] Laparoscopy has been used for both diagnostic and therapeutic purposes in penetrating abdominal trauma.[11]

Malignancy

Abdominal ultrasound, CT scan is useful in the identification of patients with advanced disease. Staging laparoscopy with laparoscopic ultrasound is less morbid than negative laparotomy. For gastric cancer, for the T stage, overall accuracy is 80% with endoscopic ultrasound (EUS) compared to 25% by CT scan.[9] EUS is ideal for T staging not for metastasis. Staging laparoscopy acts as a useful adjunct for detection of lymph nodes in gastric and esophageal malignancy.[14] Routine staging laparoscopy is recommended for hepatobiliary malignancy.[14]

REFERENCES

1. Udwadia TE. Diagnostic laparoscopy. A thirty year overview. Surg Endoscopy. 2004;18:6-10.
2. Nagy AG, et al. Diagnostic laparoscopy. Am J Surg. 1989;157:490-4.
3. Apelgren KN, et al. Laparoscopic management of gynaecologic pathologic conditions during appendectomy. Surg Clini North Am. 1996;76:487-92.

4. Diamond MP. A manual of clinical laparoscopy. New York: Parthenon; 1998.
5. Jyotsana, et al. Laparoscopic evaluation of chronic pelvic pain. vol. 14(2). JK Science, India; 2012.
6. Guidelines for diagnostic laparoscopy. Society of American Gastrointestinal Endoscopic Surgeons. Surg Endoscopy. 1993;7(4):367-8.
7. Udwadia TE, et al. Role of surgery in abdominal tuberculosis. JJJ Group Hosp. 1978;14:34-7.
8. Bailey and love. Short Practice of Surgery, 25th edition. London: Edward-Arnold Publishers Ltd; 2008. pp. 1174-5.
9. Giger U, et al. Technique and value of staging laparoscopy digestive surgery proquest health and medical complete. Dig Surg. 2002;19(6):473-8.
10. Heng –fu, et al. Value of diagnostic and therapeutic laparoscopy for abdominal stab wounds. World J Surg. 2010;34:1653-62.
11. Esposito TJ, et al. Laparoscopy in blunt trauma. 1993;34:822-8.
12. Fabian TC, et al. A prospective analysis of diagnostic laparoscopy in trauma. Ann Surg. 1993;217:557-65.
13. Demetriades D, et al. Indications for operation in abdominal stab wounds a prospective study of 651 patients. Ann Surg. 1987;205:129-32.
14. C Palanivelu. Art of Laparoscopic Surgery Textbook and Atlas. vol 1. Staging Laparoscopy in Malignancy. New Delhi: Jaypee Brothers Medical Publishers (P) Ltd; 2007. p. 127.

CHAPTER 16

Ergonomics in Laparoscopic Surgery

INTRODUCTION

The term ergonomics is derived from the Greek words "ergon" meaning work and "nomos" meaning natural laws or arrangement. Ergonomics is "the scientific study of people at work, in terms of equipment design, workplace layout, the working environment, safety, productivity, and training." Ergonomics is based on anatomy, physiology, psychology, and engineering, combined in a systems approach. In simple words, it is the science of best suiting the worker to his job, or to make the setting and surroundings favorable for the laparoscopic surgeon. The term was formally defined in 1949 and has brought benefit and safety to many areas of human endeavor.

MECHANICS AND PRINCIPAL ANGLES

Ideally the fulcrum effect should be in the middle and the instrument should be at an equal length both intra- and extracorporeally (Fig. 16.1).

Figure 16.2 represents the fulcrum near to the load arm. In this, large movements have to be made extracorporeally to produce movements intracorporeally. Also greater force is exerted at the tip of instrument, leading to tissue injury.

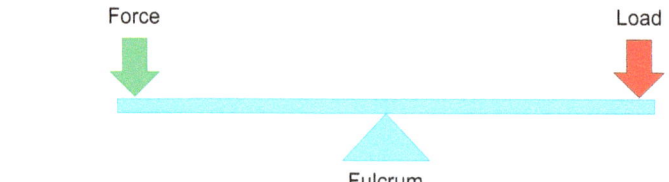

Fig. 16.1: Fulcrum middle of force and load

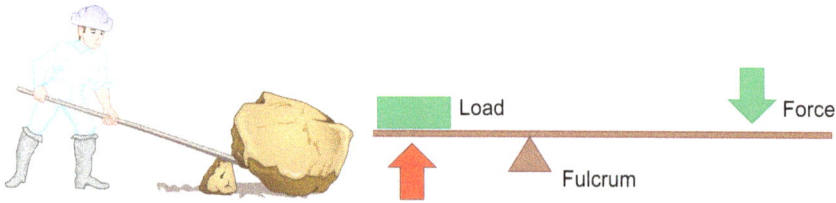

Fig. 16.2: Fulcrum near load

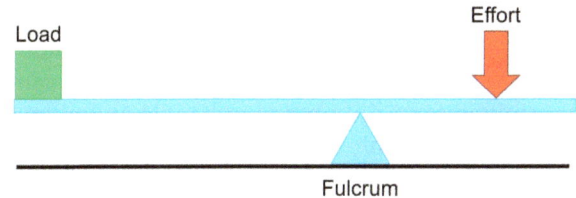

Fig. 16.3: Fulcrum near effort

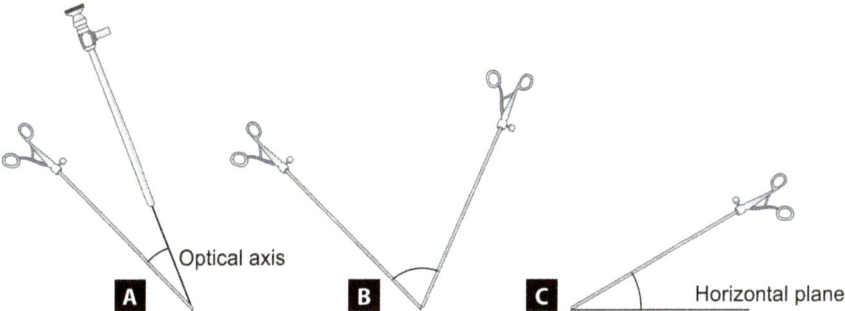

Figs 16.4A to C: (A) Azimuth angle; (B) Manipulation angle; and (C) Elevation angle

Figure 16.3 represents fulcrum near the force arm, small movements extracorporeally will produce large movements intracorporeally at the tip.

Both of which are not ideal for laparoscopic surgery.

Therefore, the instruments must be equidistance both intracorporeally and extracorporeally.

In order to prevent the stress, it is necessary to follow below-mentioned principal angles (Figs 16.4A to C).
- *Azimuth angle (30°):* The angle between telescope and operating instrument.
- *Manipulation angle (60°):* The angle formed between two operating instruments.
- *Elevation angle (60°):* The angle between instrument and body.

If the azimuth angle is >45° then there will strain in shoulder joints of the operating surgeons shoulder joints. If the angle is <30°, there will be swording action between the instruments.

Manipulation angle should be <60°. If it is >60°, there will be strain at the shoulder joint.

If elevation angle is >60°, it is not feasible for any operation. If elevation angle is <30°, it causes difficulty in operation, contact with target tissue will be lost, and extracorporeal part of the instrument will touch the anterior abdominal wall.

INSTRUMENTS

In open surgery, the thumb and the fingers exert the forces simultaneously in opposing directions. The laparoscopic instruments have pistol grip with rings for both thumb and the fingers, the force to open and close the jaws is done by the thumb alone. The thumb ring is usually located on the mobile ring of the instrument. The remaining finger ring is fixed, as the instrument is activated, the force is transmitted from thumb ring to handle and ultimately to tip of the instrument. Poor ergonomic design of the laparoscopic instruments is countered by adapting the nearest joint and limb. This relieves fatigue in group of muscles.

The palmar grip technique enables a more powerful grip, this grip uses the deep forearm flexors instead the thenar and hypothenar muscles. This decreases the fatigue of the muscles of the hand.

The standard length of the instruments in adults is 360 mm, in neonates the length of the instruments is 200 mm, in pediatrics the length of the instruments is 280 mm, and in morbidly obese, it is 450 mm.

PRINCIPLES OF PORT PLACEMENT

The first thing that strikes our mind when starting laparoscopic surgery is the position of the port. It is a well-established thing that the primary port is placed at the umbilicus as this is the thinnest portion of the abdominal wall. This port can be placed either by an open or closed method (Veress needle).

For placing the secondary ports, two circles are drawn keeping target at center, inner circle at a distance of 18 cm from target and the outer circle at a distance of 24 cm. Secondary ports are placed within the green area as shown in the circle (Fig. 16.5).

If the port is placed within the circle, then the port will be very near to the target area and large length of the instrument remains extracorporeal, and large movements at the operating hand have to be made small effects at the target of dissection. There is possibility that the uninsulated effector part

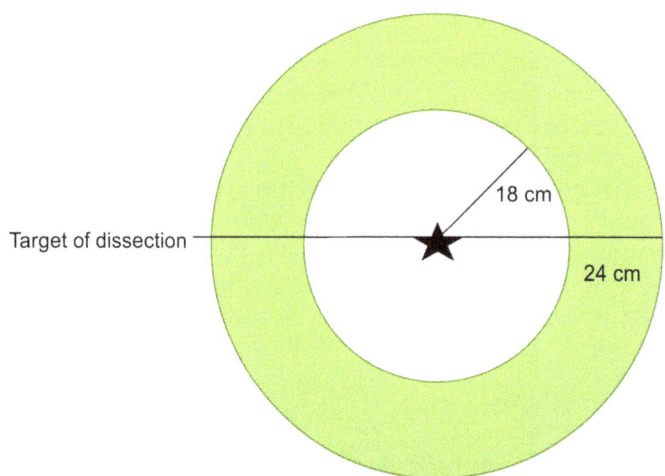

Fig. 16.5: Green area indicates area for port placements

Ergonomics in Laparoscopic Surgery

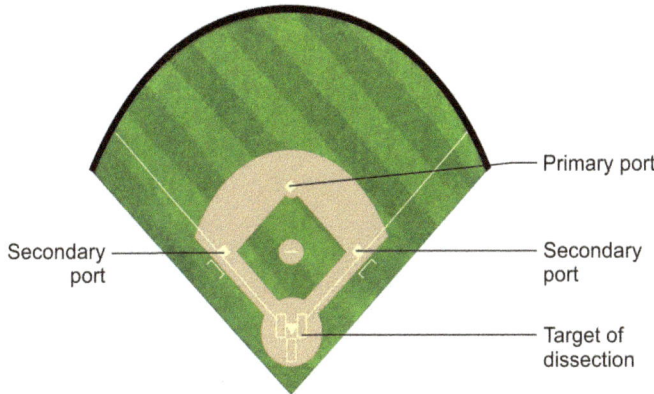

Fig. 16.6: Baseball diamond concept in laparoscopic surgery

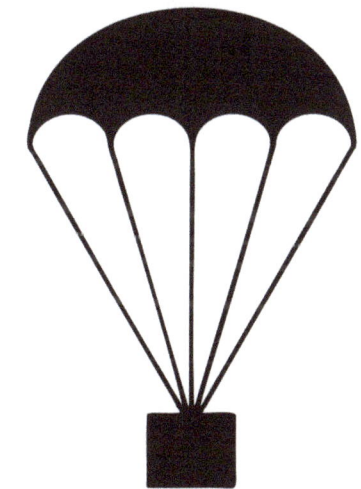

Fig. 16.7: Parachute concept in laparoscopic surgery

of the instrument may come in contact with the trocar and cause coupling injury to the vital organs.

If the port is outside the outer circle, then it will be difficult to reach the target organ. Small movements at the operating hand will produce large movements at the target of dissection.

In a 0° scope, the optical axis aligns with the physical axis of the telescope (Figs 16.6 to 16.8). Whereas in a 30° scope, the optical axis makes a 30° with the physical axis of the telescope (Fig. 16.9).

OPERATING ROOM ENVIRONMENTS[1]

Distractions and interruptions to surgical workflow are defined as an event of visible pause in the work of the surgeons or one of the team members.[1]

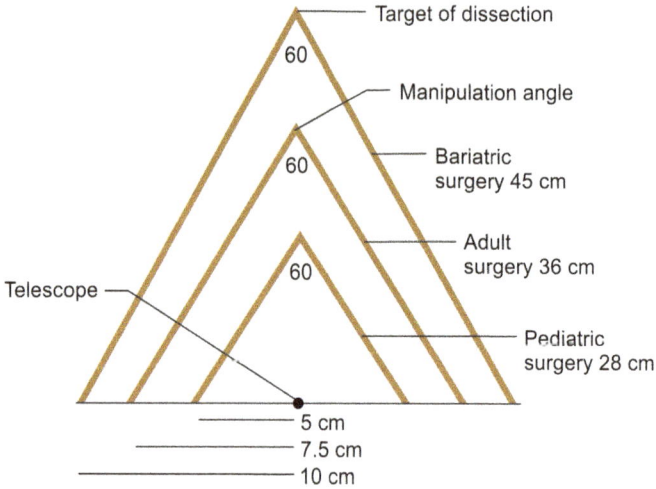

Fig. 16.8: Placement of instrument and telescope with different age group patients in laparoscopic surgery

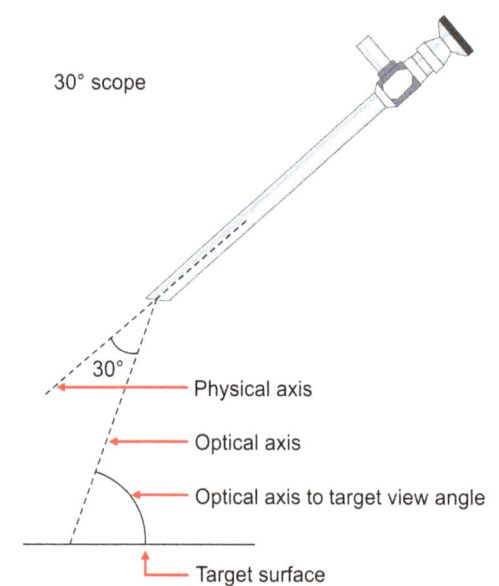

Fig. 16.9: Placement of optical axis, physical axis, and target surface in laparoscopic surgery

Psychological burdens of laparoscopic surgeons are higher than open surgeons. Minimal access surgery is more demanding and requires more concentration than open surgery, both stress and fatigue affect the surgical team in less time than open surgery. This leads to surgical fatigue syndrome manifested by exhaustion, irritability, impaired surgical judgment, and reduced dexterity.

Laparoscopic surgery entails a limited range of movements, which leads to acquire static, forced, and awkward long-term postures. The primary risk factor for appearing of musculoskeletal disorders is body deviation from neutral position.[2]

Apart from the laparoscopic monitor, the operative room should be kept in a dim to no light setting, in order to adequately expose the operating field.[1]

Monitors should be ceiling mounted and adjustable. The common problem that the surgeons face is the extension of the neck which is not ergonomically safe. The optimal position for gaze-down viewing should be 15° neck down. This is to prevent overextension of neck.[1]

Additional ceiling mounted monitor to be provided for the assistant surgeons and the nurses.

Table height is 30–60 cm (adjustable range for MIS) which allows adequate range of movements.[1]

Optimal position of arm is slight abduction, retroversion, and inward rotation. Elbow should be flexed from 90 to 120°. Intermittent relaxation of hands is advised in order to prevent fatigue.[3]

Hand activated controls for diathermy and ultrasonic energy sources are advised in order to prevent task disruption.[3]

Trunk should not be flexed >20° to avoid backache.[4]

REFERENCES

1. Soper NJ, Scott-Conner CEH. The SAGES Manual, 3rd edition. New York: Springer; 2012.
2. Sánchez-Margallo FM, Sánchez-Margallo JA. Ergonomics in laparoscopic surgery. In: Malik A (Eds). Laparoscopic Surgery. United Kingdom: IntechOpen; 2017.
3. Supe AN, Kulkarni GV, Supe PA. Ergonomics in laparoscopic surgery. J Minim Access Surg. 2010;6(2):31-6.
4. Yurteri-Kaplan LA, Park AJ. Surgical Ergonomics and Preventing Work-Related Musculoskeletal Disorders. Obstet Gynecol. 2023;141(3):455-62.

CHAPTER 17

Endotrainer

INTRODUCTION

Training in minimal access surgery has always been difficult in developing countries due to limited resources, nonavailability of formal skill laboratories and lack of trained endosurgeon, to help trainees.[1] Intracorporeal knotting and suturing are essential components for laparoscopic surgery. To improve psychomotor skills and dexterity, box training is essential.[2] Surgeons may have seen the procedure but not actually performed or assisted to understand the difference of two-dimensional (2D) vision and haptics. Several endotrainers available with varying shapes are very costly and it will be difficult for the budding surgeons and trainees. In the quest for cheaper endotrainer, we have developed our own endotrainer where the visual system (camera and monitor) can be forgone.[3] Making the roof and two sides with transparent material, in this situation there is no requirement for the visual system. The device is simple, cheap, custom made, easily portable, and nonenergy consuming. Thus, it enables to practice laparoscopic skills.[4] A self-made endotrainer also inculcates self interest in practicing more and shortening the learning curve.[4]

COMPONENTS

The main components involved in our endotrainer are as follows:
- The endotrainer box[2]
- Hand instruments—needle holder, Maryland forceps, and scissors

Different shapes of endotrainer that are available are oval, body shape, turtle shape rectangular shape, etc. Our model is a rectangular-shaped. The endotrainer is rectangular in shape. There are different modalities are available. Our endotrainer is made up of transparent acrylic material on the roof, trainee side, and other sides being opaque. The length of the endotrainer should be 250 mm, breadth should be 300 mm, and height should be 150 mm. The camera port is in the center and the working ports are on the either side of the camera at a distance of 7.5 cm, so that the angle of manipulation will be 60° at the tip of the working end. Port placements are in accordance to baseball diamond concept of laparoscopic surgery, adequate, manipulation angle, and elevation angle are also taken into consideration. Port sites are premade at the top at a distance of 5 cm from the edges of the endotrainer.

Two more port sites are made at the surgeon's side at a distance of 5 cm from the base of the endotrainer. At least two surfaces should be transparent, one being the top and the other toward the trainee. The top of the endotrainer can be open and closed from one side as it fixed by hinges on the other side. This is to facilitate to keep the suturing pad and suture material inside the endotrainer.

The suture pad is placed on an elevated slopping platform, which slopes toward the trainee. It can also be fixed to the roof to allow practice of advanced laparoscopic skills. Suture pad has three layers which replicates the texture and toughness of the skin. It is realistic, durable, and reusable making it cost-effective

SUTURING EXERCISES

The length of the suturing material should be about 15–20 cm as a longer length creates difficulty in handling the suture material. The needle length should be 20–30 mm.

ENDOTRAINER EXERCISES

- Suturing (Fig. 17.1A)
- Knotting (Fig. 17.1B)
- Ball dropping (Fig. 17.2)
- Block arranging (Fig. 17.3)
- Paper cutting (Fig. 17.4)
- Thread passing (Fig. 17.5)

While surgical simulators are being produced in ever increasing numbers, there is confusion on how to use simulators to learn the skills, so there is a need to make training objective and competency based. The conventional endotrainers are nontransparent, which necessitates the need for a visual system (webcam and monitor).

The cardboard endotrainer uses a mobile camera and mobile screen as a monitor system enabling a 2D vision and necessitating the use of

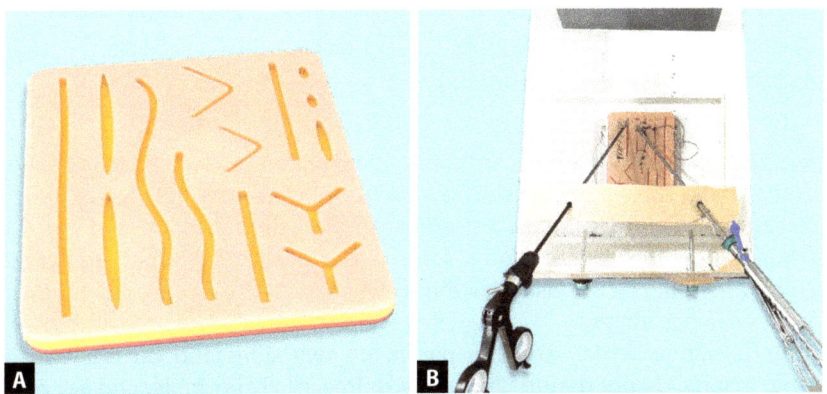

Figs 17.1A and B: (A) Suturing; (B) Knotting

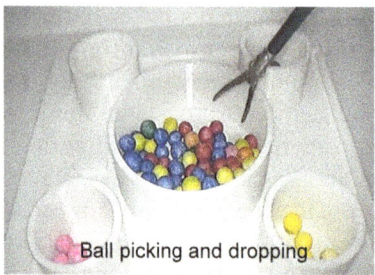

Fig. 17.2: Ball dropping

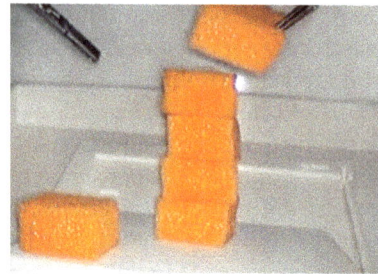

Fig. 17.3: Block arranging

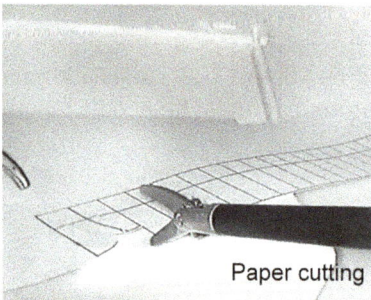

Fig. 17.4: Paper cutting

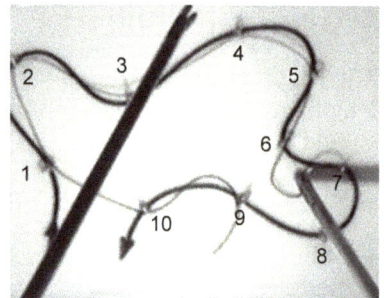

Fig. 17.5: Thread passing

Table 17.1: Differences between cardboard, conventional, and our types of endotrainer

Contents	Cardboard endotrainer	Conventional endotrainer	Our endotrainer
Monitor and webcam	Mobile phone screen	Wall mounted monitor	Not required
Hand eye coordination	Detached	Detached	Maintained
Roof	Nontransparent	Nontransparent	Transparent
Portability	Portable	Nonportable	Easily portable
Source of energy	Required	Required	Not required
Durability	Nondurable	Durable	Durable
Cost-effectiveness	Cost-effective	Expensive	Cost-effective

electrical source. The use of cardboard offers pliability at the port holes, but the lifespan of the materials used (cardboard and thermocol) is short. Though the cardboard endotrainer is cost-effective, it has not taken into account the cost of the mobile visualization system. In comparison with that our acrylic endotrainer offers a 3D vision, without the need of any electrical source, no visual system is offered.

Endotrainers which are transparent on two sides and do not have a visual system, do not require an energy source, easily portable, and are cost-effective, especially useful for young budding surgeons (Table 17.1).

REFERENCES

1. Mir IS, Mohsin M, Malik A, Shah AQ, Majid T. A structured training module using an inexpensive endotrainer for improving the performance of trainee surgeons. Trop Doct. 2008;38(4):217-8.
2. Dhariwal AK, Prabhu RY, Dalvi AN, Supe AN. Effectiveness of box trainers in laparoscopic training. J Minim Access Surg. 2007;3(2):57-63.
3. Ramalingam M, Senthil K, Murugesan A, Pai MG. Cost reductive laparoendoscopic single site surgery endotrainer and animal lab training-our methodology. Diagn Ther Endosc. 2010;2010:598165.
4. Shankar R, Madan A, Musthafa N, Kasturi S. Mobile Cam Lap Endotrainer. J Clin Diagn Res. 2016;10(7):PL03-PL04.

Index

Page numbers followed by *f* refer to figure.

A

Abdomen 87
Abdominal wall
   lower part of 31*f*
   uniform distension of 31*f*, 32*f*
Acalculous cholecystitis 75
Adhesiolysis 90
Adhesions 74*f*, 80*f*
Adnexal torsion 87
Air 28
Allis forceps 16, 16*f*
Alveolar gas
   exchange 27
   volume 25
Amplitude modulation 36*f*
Anchor-shaped secure strap 22*f*
Anorexia 61
Anterior abdominal wall 91*f*
   anatomy of 30
Appendectomy, laparoscopic 60, 63, 63*f*, 65
Appendicitis 60, 87
Appendicular artery 60
Appendix 65*f*
   anatomy of 60
   positions of 60*f*
   stump of 65*f*
Argon 29
Artery
   clip application of 81
   identification of 81
Ascites 87
Aspiration 32
Axillary port, anterior 78*f*
Azimuth angle 95, 95*f*

B

Babcock's forceps 16, 16*f*
Ball dropping 101, 102*f*
Barium meal 90
Bertram Bernheim 2
Bile duct, common 79, 83*f*
Bipolar vessel sealing device 45
Bladder injury 57
Blood pressure 27
Blunt tip 18, 19*f*
Bowel
   holding forceps 16, 16*f*
   injury 41*f*, 57
Burns, alternate site 39

C

Cable, handpiece end of 44*f*
Calcium, deposition of 72
Calot's triangle 81, 67, 78, 81, 81*f*
   dissection of 81
Camera 7, 7*f*
   control unit 7
Cannula 17, 18, 18*f*-20*f*, 65*f*
Carbon dioxide 24, 26, 28
   production 27
Cardboard endotrainer 102
Cavity
   abdominal 47
   peritoneal 31*f*, 85*f*
Charge-coupled device 7
Cholecystectomy 67, 74
   history of 76
   laparoscopic 76, 77, 77*f*
Cholecystitis
   acute 73, 74, 80*f*
   chronic 71, 73
Cholecystokinin 69
Cholesterol 71
   solubility 71
Circuit 36
Circular stapler 51, 54*f*
Clip applicator 19, 21*f*
   handle of 21*f*
   jaws of 21*f*
Closed technique 30
Coaxial handles 17
Computed tomography scan 19, 71, 92
Conical sleeve 20*f*
Conical tip 18, 19*f*

Conventional endotrainer 102
Corpus luteal cyst, ruptured 88
Creating luft-tamponade, apparatus for 3f
Current 36
   frequency of 36f
   voltage of 37f
Curved circular stapler 53f
Curved scissor 15, 15f
Cystic artery 67, 82f
   isolation 82f
Cystic duct 68f, 74f, 75f, 83f
   anomalies of 67
   clip application of 81
   identification of 81

D

Delta gap 50
Denaturation 37
Desiccation 38
Diagnostic laparoscopy 87, 87f
Diathermy generator, front panel of 37f
Direct trocar insertion 30, 32
Dismantled laparoscopic hand instrument 15f
Disposable cannula 20f
Disposable trocar 18f
   optical view of 18f
Dissection 74f, 80f, 81
Distal fallopian tube, torsion of 65f
Drain 84
Drop test 32

E

Eccentric tip 18
Echelon roticulator 52, 53f
Ectopic pregnancy 62, 87, 88
Edema, subserous 73
Electric cable 43f
   generator end of 43f
Electric circuit 10
Electrocardiogram 39f
Electrocautery 36
Elevation angle 95, 95f
Emphysema, subcutaneous 58
Endoanchor 22
Endoloop 49, 50f, 64f
   application of 49
Endoscopic linear cutter 52f, 53f
   flex roticulator knob 52f
Endoscopic ultrasound 92

Endotrainer 100, 102
   box 100
   exercises 101
Epigastric port 78f
Ergonomics 47, 94
Erich Mühe 5
Extracorporeal knots 50

F

Falciform ligament 78f
Fever 73
Fibrous form 89
Filament 9
Flap valve 18, 20f
Foot peda 44f
Forced expiratory
   flow 26
   volume 26
Forced inspiratory flow 26
Forced vital capacity 26
Forceps 16
Francois Dubois 5
Fulcrum 94f
Fulguration 38
Functional residual capacity 25

G

Gallbladder 67, 73, 73f, 74, 80f, 82, 83f-85f
   anatomy of 67
   extraction of 84, 85f
   function 69
   identifying fundus of 79f
   inflammation of 75
   large-sized solitary stone of 85f
   lymphatics of 67
   main function of 69
   mucocele of 80f
   neck of 82f
   physiology of 67
   specimen of 85f
   surgical
      anatomy of 67
      physiology of 69
Gallstone, acoustic shadowing of 72f
Gastroenteritis 62
Georg Kelling 1, 2f
German Surgical Society Anniversary Award 77
Grasper 15f

H

Halogen lamp 10, 10f
Hand grip 14f
   mechanism of 13f

Hand instruments 100
Handpiece 44*f*
   effector end of 44*f*
Hans Christian Jacobaeus 1, 2*f*
Harmonic
   and vessel sealing device 43
   devices, benefits of 45
   generator 44*f*
   scalpel 43
Harold Hopkins 4
Hartmann's pouch 67, 85*f*
Hasson cannula 34, 34*f*
Hasson sleeve 20*f*
Hasson trocar 18, 20*f*
Heinz Kalk 2, 3*f*
Helium 28
Hepatic duct 68*f*
   common 68, 68*f*
Hernia, incisional 58
Homeostasis 47
Hook scissors 15
Hypertrophic ileocecal tuberculosis 90

I

Ideal instrument, features of 14
Ideal insufflating agents 27
Ideal return pad 41
Ileal lymphatics, hypertrophy of 62
Ileitis
   regional 62
   terminal 87
Iliac fossa 33*f*, 61, 63*f*
Immunological effects 28
Incandescent bulbs 9
Infertility 87, 88
Inflamed appendix 64*f*
Inspiratory reserve volume 25
Inspiratory vital capacity 25
Instillation 32
Instruments 13
   jaws of 14
   laparoscopic 13, 15*f*
   placement of 98*f*
   tray 14*f*
Insufflating tube 24*f*
Insufflator 24, 24*f*, 25*f*
Insulation 17
   failure 40, 40*f*
Intra-abdominal pressure 25*f*
Intracorporeal knotting 49
Intussusception 62

Irrigation 20
   apparatus 20
Isolated electrosurgical system 39, 40*f*

J

Janos Veress 4

K

Knotting 101
Kurt Semm 2, 3*f*, 63*f*

L

Laparoscope 8
Laparoscopy 7, 26*f*, 56, 56, 76, 92
   beginning of 1
   complications of 57
   unit 13*f*
LigaSure 45
Light source 9, 9*f*
Liver
   disease 87, 88
   floppy left lobe of 85
   tumors 87, 89
Lower midline scar 33*f*
Lymph node 81*f*
   dissection 81*f*
Lymphoid hyperplasia 60

M

Magnetic resonance imaging 19
Malignancy 92
Manipulation angle 95, 95*f*
Maryland forceps 16, 16*f*
Mass abdomen 87
McBurney's point 61, 61*f*
Meckel's diverticulitis 62, 87
Mesenteric adenitis 62, 87
Mesoappendix 60
   dissection of 64*f*
Metal oxide semiconductor device 7
Microtip scissors 15
Midclavicular port 79*f*
Midline scar 33*f*
Minimal access surgery 98, 100
Mittelschmerz disease 62
Modern insufflators 24
Monitors 11
   specifications 12

Monopolar
    diathermy, circuit of 39*f*
    electrosurgery 38
    energy 37
Movement 32
Murphy's sign 73
Muscles 30
Mycobacterium tuberculosis 90

N

National Institute of Health 5
Nausea 61, 73
Needle
    holder 16, 47
    loading of 48
    types of 48*f*
Nitrous oxide 29
Nodules 89*f*

O

Obturator 20*f*
    sign 62
Oddi sphincter 69
Ohm's law 37
Omental adhesions 80*f*
Omentum 61
Open appendectomy 65
Open technique 30, 34
Operating room environments 97
Optical
    axis, placement of 98*f*
    fiber cable 12*f*
    trocar insertion 30
Optics, principle of 11*f*
Outer sheath, self-adjusting seal of 19*f*
Ovarian cyst
    hemorrhage of 62
    ruptured 87
    torsion of 62

P

Pain
    abdominal 87, 88
    periumbilical 61
    shifting of 61
Palmer's point 33*f*, 87, 92
Palmer's technique 34, 96
Paper cutting 101, 102*f*
Peak expiratory flow 26
Pelvic
    appendix 62
    inflammatory disease 87
    pain 88

Perforated peptic ulcer 62
Peritoneal access 30
    methods of 30
Peritoneum 30, 89*f*
Philippe Mouret 4, 5*f*
Physical axis, placement of 98*f*
Pigment stones 71
Pneumomediastinum 58
Pneumoperitoneum 24, 25, 30
    insufflation 26
Pneumothorax 58
Pointing sign 61
Porcelain gallbladder 72
Port
    placement 96*f*
        principle of 96
    position 77, 78*f*
    site, infection of 58
Processor 7*f*
Psoas sign 62
Purulent form 89
Pyramidal tip obturator 18, 19*f*
Pyrexia 61

R

Raoul Palmer 4
Rectus
    abdominis muscle 30
    sheath hematoma 62
Reducer 19, 20*f*, 21*f*
Return electrode 41
    correct placement of 41*f*
    incorrect placement of 41*f*
Right distal salpinx following tubectomy,
        torsion of 88*f*
Right-angled forceps 15*f*
    dissecting cystic duct 83*f*
Roeder's knot 50*f*
Rovsing's sign 61

S

Salpingitis 62, 87
Saw-toothed forceps 16*f*
Scissors 14, 15*f*
Semm's electronic insufflator 3*f*
Serrated scissors 15
Skin fascia 30
Sleeve reducer 21*f*
Society of American Gastrointestinal
        Surgeons 6, 76
Spatula 15, 15*f*
Spring-loaded stylet 22*f*

Square knot 49
Staple configuration 51*f*
Stapler 50
    removal of 55*f*
Stone 73*f*, 85*f*
Straight forceps 16, 16*f*
Straight scissor 15, 15*f*
Subcoastal scar 33*f*
Suction 20
    apparatus 21*f*
    handle of 21*f*
    irrigation system 20
Surgery, laparoscopic 58, 91, 94, 97*f*, 98*f*, 99
Suturing 101
    exercises 101
    material 47
    technique 47

T

Telescope 8*f*
    interiors of 9*f*
    tip, cleaning of 9*f*
Tenderness 61
Tidal volume 25
Total internal reflection 11, 11*f*
Total lung capacity 25
Transverse abdominis muscles 30
Trauma 87, 92
Trocar 17, 18*f*, 33*f*
    description of 17*f*
    outer sheath of 17*f*
Troubleshooting 56
Trumpet valve 18
Tubal pregnancy 88
Tubectomy 65*f*
Tubercular abdomen 89*f*
Tuberculosis
    abdominal 90*f*
    intestinal 90
    peritoneal 89

Tuberculous mesenteric lymphadenitis 90
Tubo-ovarian mass 62
Tumor staging 87
Tungsten filament 10
Twist 50, 51*f*

U

Ulcerative ileocecal tuberculosis 90
Ultrasonic shears 44
Ultrasound, abdominal 92
Umbilical port 78*f*, 87
Umbilicus 30, 33*f*, 61*f*, 87
Upper midline scar 33*f*
Ureteric colic 62
U-shaped
    configuration 23
    secure strap 23*f*

V

Valve 18, 19*f*
    outer sheath of 17*f*
Vascular injury 57
Veress needle 22, 22*f*, 30, 31, 31*f*-33*f*, 34, 63, 87
    closed valve of 31*f*
    spring action of 30*f*
    stylet of 32*f*
    technique 30
Veress outer sheath 22*f*
Vicryl 47
Vital capacity 25
Vomiting 61, 73

W

Weaning 62

X

Xenon arc light 9*f*

EU GSPR Authorised Reprsentative
Logos Europe, 9 rue Nicolas Poussin
1700, La Rochelle, France
Phone: +33 (0) 6 67 93 73 78
E-mail: contact@logoseurope.eu

www.ingramcontent.com/pod-product-compliance
Ingram Content Group UK Ltd.
Pitfield, Milton Keynes, MK11 3LW, UK
UKHW051846210426